WOMEN, POWER,
AND
CHILDBIRTH

WOMEN, POWER,
AND
CHILDBIRTH

A Case Study of a
Free-Standing Birth Center

Kathleen Doherty Turkel

BERGIN & GARVEY
Westport, Connecticut • London

Library of Congress Cataloging-in-Publication Data

Turkel, Kathleen Doherty.
   Women, power, and childbirth : a case study of a free-standing
  birth center / Kathleen Doherty Turkel.
      p.   cm.
  Includes bibliographical references and index.
  ISBN 0–89789–317–4 (alk. paper)
   1. Birthing centers—United States—Case studies. 2. Childbirth—
Social aspects—United States. 3. Childbirth—Political aspects—
United States. I. Title.
RG500.T87 1995
362.1′982′00973—dc20   95–12839

British Library Cataloguing in Publication Data is available.

Library of Congress Catalog Card Number: 95–12839
ISBN: 0–89789–317–4

First published in 1995

Bergin & Garvey, 88 Post Road West, Westport, CT 06881
An imprint of Greenwood Publishing Group, Inc.

Printed in the United States of America

The paper used in this book complies with the
Permanent Paper Standard issued by the National
Information Standards Organization (Z39.48–1984).

10 9 8 7 6 5 4 3 2 1

In Memory of My Grandmothers

Helen Rucinski Grodzicki
and
Anne Green Doherty

Contents

Acknowledgments

There are many people whose cooperation, assistance, and support helped to make this book possible. I would like to thank all of those involved with the birth center which I studied and of which I continue to be a part. There are particular individuals whose dedication to the birth center project and to the center's clients make this wonderful place and the birth experiences it offers possible. There are others whose work in the larger community promotes and supports the rights of childbearing women. My interest in maintaining their anonymity prevents me from identifying them by name. However, I would like to offer my sincerest thanks for the work they do and for the important contributions they have made to my research.

The help of Robert Warren was invaluable to me in doing the early research which resulted in this book. In addition, I would like to thank Dan Rich, Kate Conway-Turner, and the late Anne Mooney for their direction and advice.

Linda Keen's skill, precision, and good humor were extremely important in preparing the manuscript. She went far beyond the call of duty and I appreciate it. I would like to extend special thanks to Suzanne Solensky and Deborah Ross for their skillful editing and production assistance.

I am also grateful to my children, Eli and Helen, for being constant sources of joy and for helping to keep things in perspective. They are reminders of the importance of research on childbirth. Finally, and most important, I would like to thank my husband, Gerry Turkel. His criticisms of early drafts of the manuscript were invaluable. He is an unwavering source of intellectual, emotional, and physical support.

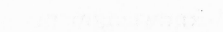

1

Introduction

As Adrienne Rich reminds us, birth—the experience of being born of woman—is the one unifying experience shared by all people. Birth is a supremely human, intensely intimate event, the effects of which we carry throughout our lives (Rich, 1986). But birth is also a cultural event. As such it reflects dominant cultural beliefs and values. Beliefs about birth and the practices which surround birth can tell us about power relations within a society and about how a society views technology. They can also tell us a great deal about gender, race, and class.

My interest in childbirth initially grew out of a general interest in women's health and health policy. I was in California during the summer of 1978 when lay midwife Marianne Doshi was charged with manslaughter and practicing medicine without a license. Doshi was unable to resuscitate a newborn infant whose birth she was attending. An ambulance was called. Ambulance attendants revived the child and she was transported to a hospital, where she died shortly after admittance. The parents who had lost their child were not interested in bringing charges against Doshi. They were satisfied that she had acted competently and had done as much as anyone could have under the circumstances. The district attorney pursued the charges, but ultimately they were dismissed by Judge Richard C. Kirkpatrick, who said, "I am convinced from reading [the medical testimony] that had the child died in the hospital or at home under a doctor's care, that we would have had a thousand doctors lined up between here and Los Angeles willing to testify that the doctor provided medical treatment according to the standard of care" (Ruzek, 1980, p. 346).

In reflecting upon this case, I realized that I had never given much thought to the medical model of birth or to alternatives to it. I knew that in the 1930s, my grandmother had given birth to three sets of twins at home with the assistance of a midwife. I also knew that my own mother had suffered a severe case of toxemia at the end of her pregnancy with me in the early 1950s. Toxemia, a disease which occurs only during pregnancy, is characterized by edema (swelling), a rise in blood pressure, and the presence of protein in the urine. An incompetent doctor had failed to recognize the severity of her condition. My grandmother who had birthed three sets of twins was the one who recognized the danger my mother was in and insisted that she be hospitalized. My father's aunt was a nurse at the hospital to which my mother was admitted. She was dissatisfied with the way my mother's doctor was handling her care and insisted that another doctor be called in on the case. This doctor performed an emergency Cesarean section. The doctor, however, is not the hero of this story. The heroes, to me, are my mother for her bravery and endurance in the face of horribly incompetent care and advice, my grandmother for her wisdom in trusting her experiential knowledge gained through birthing her own children, and my father's aunt for trusting her own judgment and recognizing that the doctor did not know best.

Despite the fact that I had grown up hearing about my grandmother's and my mother's experiences, I still accepted the idea that a high-tech, hospitalized birth was the best and the safest. It was the Doshi case which jarred me into thinking about birth more critically.

I began reading about the medical model of birth and about midwives, home birth, and free-standing birth centers. I also began talking to women about their birth experiences. I quickly rejected the idea that the medical model offered the best and safest alternative. I concluded, instead, that the medical model of birth represented nothing short of the theft of the experience of birth from women. Authors such as Jordan, Rothman, Oakley, Kitzinger, and Harrison helped to deepen my understanding of the politics surrounding childbirth. They also helped to validate my conclusions about the medical model. Nothing I have read, no one I have talked with, nothing I have experienced in over twelve years of doing research on childbirth, has in any way altered this conclusion.

A critical perspective on childbirth led me to want to know more about the legal, political, economic, and technological factors which shape childbirth options. How are dominant patterns created and maintained? More important, what are the factors which either block or facilitate the development and maintenance of patterns of childbirth which challenge the medical model?

In 1980 I began what turned out to be a long-term study of the establishment and first twelve years of operation of a free-standing birth center (FSBC). FSBCs are out-of-hospital birthing facilities which are physically and, usually, administratively separate from hospitals. The model for such centers is the home, not the hospital. A birth center is not a hospital and does not routinely use procedures and technologies which are standard in hospital births, such as Pitocin for inducing and stimulating labor, epidurals or other anesthetics, and electronic fetal heart monitoring. Birth centers are short-stay facilities. Women who give birth at birth centers stay between four and twelve hours following birth and then return home. Generally, births at FSBCs are attended by nurse-midwives. They provide prenatal care, attend women during labor and birth, and provide postnatal care. The law in about half of the states requires that nurse-midwives demonstrate written evidence of an alliance with a physician or physicians who can provide medical backup when necessary. In the rest of the states it is expected that such a collaborative arrangement with a physician will be in place.

It is important for the reader to know that the names of people directly and indirectly involved with the birth center that I studied have been changed, and references to places that might identify the birth center have been omitted. There are also references in the text to a local newspaper. In an effort to maintain the anonymity of the people involved with the birth center I do not identify the newspaper or give any specific citations for articles that appeared in the paper.

Initially, a group of consumers in the state which I studied set out to establish a consumer-run birth center with services provided by nurse-midwives. This group, which I will call "Babyplace," struggled for over a year to gain support and to find a nurse-midwife and a backup physician who would work with them. I attended meetings with Babyplace and interviewed the members to document their reasons for wanting to provide an out-of-hospital birthing facility, the problems which they encountered, and the sources of support for their efforts.

Several months after Babyplace made their intentions public, a nurse-midwife who was well known in the area announced her intentions to open a free-standing birth center. The nurse-midwife, whom I will call Anne Watson, had once been the head of parent education programs at a local medical center. She left that job following a conflict stemming from her advocacy for birthing women and became the director of nurse-midwifery service at a free-standing birth center in an adjacent state. By the early 1980s, she decided the time was right to open a birth center in her home state. I followed Anne's efforts and compared them to those of Babyplace. I was interested in whether or not they might form an alliance, how their approaches would differ, and whether Anne's status as a health professional would give her an advantage over the consumer group.

This book is the story of these two attempts to open a free-standing birth center and of Anne's eventual success. Beyond that, it is the story of some of the events during the center's twelve years of operation. To tell this story, I conducted interviews with health care providers, hospital administrators, insurance providers, health planners, and clients. I worked as a volunteer to observe the operation of the birth center and the relationships between nurse-midwives and clients. I attended public meetings and forums where the concept of out-of-hospital birthing was discussed. Eventually, I served on a consumer advisory group concerned with the loss of malpractice insurance for nurse-midwives and birth centers. I became part of a consumer board to foster public education about nurse-midwifery. I also sought the care of Anne and the other nurse-midwives at the birth center for the births of my own children.

In order to tell this story it is necessary to locate it within its larger social and cultural context. It is necessary to look at dominant conceptions of birth and to consider how these are challenged by the concept of the free-standing birth center.

The way a society conceptualizes birth is the most significant indicator of how birth will be organized and carried out in that society. In the United States, birth is defined primarily as a medical event. This is consistent with the contemporary practice in the United States of defining most physiological processes as falling within the medical domain, including issues relating to nutrition or obesity, sexual concerns, learning difficulties, and dying (Jordan, 1993, pp. 48–49).

The implications of this medical definition of birth are many. First and foremost, pregnant women are seen as "patients." Pregnancy is viewed as a "condition" requiring treatment from physicians, technicians, and nurses who make use of a variety of procedures, tests, and high-tech diagnostic tools to assess the health of the pregnant woman and of the developing fetus and the overall progress of the pregnancy. Birth itself takes place in a hospital setting under the direction of a physician and the assistance of nurses and technicians who rely upon an array of technologies to assess the progress of the event (Arney, 1982; Davis-Floyd, 1992; Eakins, 1986a; Jordan, 1993; Rothman, 1982, 1989).

When laboring women leave their homes and enter hospitals to give birth, they move into an unfamiliar domain in which they are able to exercise little control. Women I have interviewed about their hospital experiences report having to ask permission for nearly everything. They were not permitted to wear their own clothes. Physicians and hospital policy determined how many people could be there with them while they gave birth. Other children were not permitted to watch the birth. Food and drink were restricted and so was physical movement. Women describe feeling as if they had to try to be quiet and not create problems for the staff. Decision making takes place within the confines of the institutional rules and regulations and rests in the hands of medical personnel, most specifically physicians (Eakins, 1986a). The social construction of birth within U.S. hospitals privileges the technical knowledge of the physician while it discounts and ignores the experiential knowledge of birthing women (Rothman, 1982, 1989; Eakins, 1986a; Davis-Floyd, 1992; Jordan, 1993).

One justification for this high level of medical intervention is that birth is dangerous and unpredictable. High-tech medicine is needed to assure healthy babies and good outcomes. Yet there is little, if any, evidence which suggests that the routine use of existing high-tech procedures leads to better birth outcomes. In many instances, their use is counterproductive (Rothman, 1982, 1989; Davis-Floyd, 1992; Jordan, 1993). Given the availability of evidence which, at a minimum, seriously questions the appropriateness of dominant birthing procedures, a core question is why and how these dominant practices are maintained.

Since we cannot account for the routine medicalization of birth by the benefits it confers, we must consider other explanations. An answer to the question of how medical practice and medical authority in relation to birthing women are established and maintained requires an analysis which locates medical practice within its larger social and political context, and in relation to the ideologies which define it. For Rothman and other feminist scholars, the core ideologies are those of technology, patriarchy, and capitalism (Rothman, 1989; Oakley, 1986; Rich, 1986).

Major features of the technocratic approach to understanding the relationship between technology and society include (1) a belief that technological development is neutral with regard to social interests and synonymous with progress, (2) a belief that technical information and expertise should provide the grounds for decision making, and (3) a belief that efficiency, productivity, rationality, and control should serve as the standards by which we judge not only machines and organizations, but human beings as well (Kahn and Weiner, 1967; Kranzberg, 1980; Florman, 1980; Rothman, 1989).

There is little, if any, concern about economic and political power and the power disparities which exist within our society. There is also very little concern that a reliance on technical information and expertise leads to an exclusion of experiential knowledge and makes it impossible for people to participate in decisions regarding their everyday lives. The ideology of technology is not about tools and gadgets, but rather about viewing the world in mechanical-industrial terms. Evidence of the pervasiveness of this ideology in our society is the extent to which it influences our thinking even where it is not appropriate. We use mechanical metaphors to talk about the human body and human emotions. We talk about "working the bugs out" of relationships and "interfacing" with colleagues and friends. We wonder what "makes people tick." We value what we are less than what we can make (Rothman, 1989, pp. 48–50).

Beyond the ways in which technocratic and commodity thinking affects childbirth, the general subordination of women supports male domination of birthing. In a patriarchal society, motherhood remains under male control. Women have been, and continue to be, portrayed as having very little knowledge about what motherhood actually entails. Oakley argues that in the twentieth century, women's own knowledge has been characterized as inauthentic. She states, "Stripped of its internal authenticity, motherhood becomes an exercise in professional consultation, an axis of self-doubt, and a black hole into which "liberated" women disappear only to be besieged by visions of all they gave up (or never had), in order to fulfill this one great intimate destiny" (Oakley, 1986, p. 134).

The experiences of women in relation to motherhood become consumed by what Rich calls the "institution" of motherhood, that is, all of the social, political, and economic forces which define and interpret motherhood and which keep it under male control. Rich distinguishes between the institution of motherhood and the experience of motherhood, which she defines as the "potential relationship of any woman to her powers of reproduction and to children." In our society, as in many others, it is women who are responsible for children, for bearing them, for raising them, for the circumstances in which they live their lives. It is women who are accountable for the health and well-being of children (Rich, 1986, p. 13). The extent to which this is the case is demonstrated by the recent debate over infant mortality in my state.

The state in which I live has a very high infant mortality rate. In late 1994 a major newspaper in the state ran a series of articles trying to draw public attention to this problem. The articles dealt with a range of issues which the author of the series saw as contributing to infant mortality including teen pregnancy, poverty, lack of prenatal care, and drug use during pregnancy. While the series was running, the newspaper ran an editorial outlining what they thought should be done about infant mortality. The solution was simple: women need to take more responsibility. They need to be more responsible about their sexual behavior. They need to adopt more responsible lifestyles during pregnancy. They need to take better care of their children. Rich refers to this responsibility which women are called upon to accept as "powerless responsibility." Women are held responsible even though they are mothering within a political-economic context which they do not control. Mothers often face poverty, unemployment, a lack of day care, poor school systems, and violence in their streets and in their homes. Yet it is they who are responsible for the problems their children experience (Rich, 1986, p. 52).

This lack of power which the institution of motherhood implies extends to the experience of pregnancy and childbirth. Rich describes the powerlessness of giving birth in a hospital where childbirth is a feature of hierarchical organization and high technology. Women are alienated from their bodies and from the experience of giving birth to their own children.

While high technology is a defining characteristic of hospital birth, high technology is not limited to this context. It is necessary to consider the context in which this technology exists and the ideology which shapes and determines its use. The ideology of technology within the context of corporate capitalism creates new "ground rules" for public and private decision making. Decisions are rooted in cost-benefit analysis and technocratic expertise (Dickson, 1984). Economics, Wolin argues, acts as a public language which serves the needs of modern science, technology, capitalism, and the state (1981). Dominant political and economic forces not only determine the shape and use of high technology, but also control the production of scientific knowledge upon which such technology is based (Dickson, 1984).

In late capitalist society, everything is subject to commodification, including human beings. Everything can be bought and sold, including male sperm and female eggs. Graduate student Gwen Martin wrote about her experience when she considered selling some of her eggs to a fertility clinic. Martin responded to an ad which appeared in her campus newspaper. A hospital was offering $2,000 to a woman willing to donate eggs to an infertile couple. In Martin's words, "I'd never before realized I had a commodity to offer: my fertility" (1994, p. 168). When Martin contacted the hospital she was asked about her age, her menstrual cycle, and her ethnicity. They were also interested in her skin color and eye color. She was told that if she wanted to be an egg donor she would have to undergo medical examination, psychological testing, and personal interviews.

Martin decided to go ahead. She describes her treatment by the doctors and clinic staff. They were, she felt, interested in her ovaries but not in her. At one point during her participation in the program she discovered that she had been given an intelligence test without her knowledge. There was only one possible purpose for such testing in Martin's view: "to define me as a higher-or-lower-quality product in the reproductive marketplace" (1994, p. 168). As the intricacies of egg harvesting became clear to Martin, she began to have doubts about the program. She was concerned about the possible long-term effects of the hormones used to cause several eggs to ripen at once. Ultimately she felt demeaned and used. In the end she dropped out of the program before any of her eggs were removed. Examples such as Martin's demonstrate the extent to which our contemporary definitions of motherhood define babies as products. Women's bodies become defined as resources for producing babies (Rothman, 1989, p. 65).

Dominant beliefs and practices in relation to pregnancy and birth are shaped and supported by technocratic ideology, powerful economic and political resources translated into institutional and legal controls, and by a system of patriarchal power which undermines the ability of women to control their own bodies and to participate in meaningful ways in shaping the conditions of their lives. These forces have shaped the everyday understanding of birth in American culture, as well as the expectations that many women have about the physical, psychological, and emotional experience of pregnancy and birth (Rich, 1976; Rothman, 1982, 1989; Jordan, 1993; Davis-Floyd, 1992). Common conceptions about birth are that it is a risky event requiring hospitalization. High technology is required to insure the health and safety of mothers and babies. I discuss childbirth frequently in the university courses which I teach. While some students are critical of dominant birth practices, most belong to the "what if something goes wrong" school of thought. They might agree with some of the criticisms of hospital practices and procedures and they might like the idea of birth outside the hospital, but they believe that birth needs to take place in a hospital "in case something goes wrong." Hospitals have all the high-technology equipment that an emergency might require. It is the technology that is important. For the most part, these students have given very little thought to having children or to the circumstances under which they would like their children to be born, but they have internalized the values and beliefs of the medical model of birth. Birth is a risk-filled experience. The only way to minimize the risk is for birth to be hospitalized with medical experts and high-tech devices at the ready.

Despite the dominance of the medical model, there are practitioners and models of birth which challenge the dominant ideas and practices. Home birth and birth in free-standing birth centers are examples of challenges to dominant patterns which can give women more power and control over birth. Although these challenges exist, they do so within a context which undermines their existence. Those seeking to provide out-of-hospital birthing services for women face a variety of legal and institutional constraints. The nature of these constraints varies according to specific state law and to the particular political climate in any given state.

One source of constraint is the legal construction of attending birth as practicing medicine. Laws governing the practice of medicine are state laws. As a result, specific definitions of what constitutes the practice of medicine—who can and who cannot practice medicine and under what circumstances—

will vary from state to state. With respect to childbirth, physicians are recognized in every state as having the legal authority to attend women in childbirth. Home births and births in free-standing birth centers are most frequently attended by lay midwives, direct-entry midwives, or by nurse-mid-wives.

There is no unified body of law that regulates the practice of midwifery. Certified nurse-midwives can legally practice in virtually every state, but about half of all states require that they have an alliance with a physician in order to practice. There is tremendous variation in state laws which define and govern the practice of nurse-midwifery. In a number of states the practice of nurse-midwifery is authorized under the state's nurse practice act. In some of these states nurse-midwives are mentioned specifically in the statute, while in others they are not. In some states the law requires nurse-midwives to be licensed as registered nurses (RNs). Other states require a midwifery license but no RN license. In a number of states nurse-midwives have the authority to issue prescriptions. This is becoming more common as more states pass advanced practice nursing legislation which often grants such authority to nurses, including nurse-midwives. Regulating bodies for nurse-midwifery also vary by state. Nurse-midwives are regulated by the board of health in some states, while in others they are regulated by the board of nursing, the board of medical examiners, the department of professional regulators, or some combination of regulating boards. The process and frequency of license renewal also vary. In some instances there is no renewal process. In most states licenses must be renewed every one, two, or three years (Bidgood-Wilson, Barickman, and Ackley, 1992). The law is even less consistent with respect to the practice of lay midwifery and direct-entry midwifery. In some states these are legal, in other states they are illegal, and in still other states they are not mentioned in the law (Sullivan and Weitz, 1988; Sallomi, Pallow-Fleury, and McMahon, 1982).

Midwives of all kinds generally share a philosophy which sees pregnancy and birth as a healthy process, not a pathological condition. Nurse-midwives find themselves on somewhat firmer legal footing, however, because of their status as health professionals. They are nurses with graduate training in midwifery and, in most cases, certification from the American College of Nurse-Midwives. Lay midwives do not necessarily have any formal training or credentials. They learn by observing births, eventually participating as assistants, and finally becoming a primary attendant. Direct-entry midwives complete a course of training which meets requirements for state licensure in those states which license direct-entry midwives (Myers-Ciecko, 1988, p. 63).

The argument for extending legal recognition to lay midwifery and to direct-entry midwifery rests on the definition of childbirth as a healthy process rather than as a pathological one. If this definition is accepted, attending women in childbirth would not be viewed as the practice of medicine. Indeed, the question of how childbirth is defined is at the center of the debate over the power of the medical profession in relation to childbirth. As long as childbirth is viewed as a medical event requiring hospitalization and technology to be accomplished, physicians can continue to exercise a virtual monopoly over attending women in childbirth and over defining standards of treatment in relation to birthing. Locating birth within the hospital has been a primary factor in the creation and maintenance of this monopoly, because "hospitalization of childbirth is the medium through which the philosophy of interventive obstetrics is carried into practice" (Tew, 1990, p. 20).

Although women-centered birthing options are available, technological developments and the interests of the medical profession continue to usurp control over birth from women. Even when the motivation for establishing out-of-hospital childbirth services is to assert the reproductive rights of women and the value of their experiences, such practices may still be absorbed into the institutional framework and logic of the dominant model. Arney (1982) has argued, for example, that the limits to the discourse on childbirth alternatives are determined by the profession of obstetrics. DeVries (1985) believes that nurse-midwives and licensed lay midwives are under pressure to accommodate to the medical model. Woman-centered approaches to birth remain marginal to the medical model, which to a large extent shapes and defines them culturally and even legally.

The medical model of birth focuses on those factors which can be measured and technologically managed, most notably mortality and morbidity rates. Many authors have pointed out that in-hospital and planned out-of-hospital births fare about the same when judged by these measures. Others would argue that out-of-hospital births fare better (Rothman, 1989, 1982). But there are other factors which are not so easily measured which are equally important. Birth is an important personal and family event. Indeed, it is life altering. The experience of birth extends far beyond the event itself and affects not only mothers and babies, but fathers, siblings, extended family members, and friends.

In trying to put into words those immeasurable but crucially important things about birth, Michelle Harrison asks:

> What do we need to know about a birth? What are we missing when we score a baby by heartbeats per minute? What are the questions we should be asking as we try to describe the emergence of one human being out of the body of another?

Was there awe?

Do those in the room feel close to each other and the baby?

Does this baby look healthy?

Does this baby feel welcomed into the world?

Does the baby make eye contact?

Is the baby curious?

Does the baby respond to touch, to voice, to being held?

What is the mother's mood? Happy? Depressed? Frightened?

What is the baby's mood? Happy? Depressed? Frightened?

Was the baby smiling in the birth canal?

Does this mother feel good about herself after this birth?

Is the mother ready to move on to the next phase of their relationship, whether that is together or apart?

Was love present? (Harrison, 1982, pp. 85–86)

To me, the experience of birth, unencumbered by unnecessary machines, medication, or health professionals who interfere rather than support, is as good as life gets. I am always mystified when those of us who argue in favor of alternatives to the medical model of birth are characterized, as we were in an editorial in the *Wall Street Journal* on November 6, 1992, as masochistic feminists who prefer to act as martyrs rather than to be spared the painful parts of birth through the array of drugs and paraphernalia available. Pain is, indeed, part of labor and birth for most women. But it is only part of the process. Pain is part of many human activities which involve physical exertion. When drugs are used to dull the pain of birth, the pain may be dulled (but not necessarily), but so is everything else. The rest of what birth is becomes lost in the process.

Recently Anne Watson, director of the birth center which I studied, asked birth center clients to consider why they chose to experience the pain of labor when it is possible to eliminate it. She asked them to put some of their thoughts in writing. Some women talked about the negative effects of drugs and other aspects of the medical model. These are important and have been discussed a great deal in the literature. But the accounts which I found most moving were the ones which talked about what is gained through the experience of birth. One anonymous woman wrote:

After twenty-two hours of slow labor (slow, but progressive), I wanted no more of it. *No more. Take me to the hospital and give me drugs.* My midwife wrapped her arms around me and whispered in my ear. You can do this. Women have been doing this forever, and you can, too. And when you do, you will know that you have the power to achieve anything. And, when my son was born that early spring morning—the birds were singing. I can still hear the birds!—I was born with him. I emerged from that profound experience a stronger person, more confident, more alive than I have ever been before.

These comments represent what birth should be, a positive, empowering experience for women, for their children, and for anyone else involved. A fundamental concern of this book is how approaches to birth which empower women can be created and maintained.

Since the mid-1970s we have seen the establishment of free-standing birth centers. To what extent do free-standing birth centers provide an alternative to the medical model, and to what extent are they dependent upon this model? Through empirical research it becomes possible to specify the concrete social, economic, and technological relations which shape the medical model of birth and the approaches which challenge it.

In what follows I discuss the context in which a free-standing birth center was established. I look at the process and politics involved in establishing the birth center, and I discuss its operation. Chapter 2 discusses technocratic ideology and its role in shaping our contemporary cultural beliefs about medicine in general and childbirth in particular. Chapter 3 analyzes the assumptions of the medical model of birth and the dominant childbirth practices and procedures which this model dictates. In Chapter 4, I examine the challenge to the medical model posed by the midwifery approach and present the philosophy which this approach represents. I also discuss some of the difficulties faced by midwives in the face of the power of the medical model. In Chapter 5 I look at the concept of the free-standing birth center.

Chapters 6 through 8 focus on the establishment and operation of the birth center. In Chapter 6, I discuss the two attempts to establish a birth center and why one was eventually successful. In Chapter 7, I discuss the facility which was established, the day-to-day operation of the center, and the clientele. Chapter 8 looks at the realities of running an FSBC within an institutional and cultural context dominated by established medical interests. Chapter 9 includes concluding thoughts and speculates about the future of FSBCs.

2

Technocratic Ideology and the Medical Marginalization of Motherhood and Birth

How can one be pessimistic about something called "technology"? This is like being pessimistic about art or science, or music, or government or religion. It is possible to be pessimistic only about the use that human beings will make of technology. But this is to say that one is pessimistic about humankind—pessimistic about *life*—and such a remark is childish.
—Samuel C. Florman, "Technology and the Tragic View," p. 24

TECHNOCRATIC PERSPECTIVES

Underlying views of science and technology buttress and rationalize dominant medical practice toward birth. As such, these views of science and technology must be confronted and critiqued in order to reveal the ways in which the medicalization of birth has appropriated women's experience and power. In this chapter, I critique approaches to science and technology as ideology from critical theory and feminist perspectives. This makes it possible to see how technocratic ideology shapes dominant birth practice.

In their 1967 essay, "The Next Thirty Years: Framework for Speculation," Kahn and Weiner presented a classic argument for linking human progress to high technology. The authors identified one hundred areas in which they believed technological innovation would occur before the year 2000. The authors admitted that some items on their list were controversial. These include:

- More extensive use of transplantation of human organs
- New techniques in the education of children

- New kinds of very cheap, convenient, and reliable birth-control techniques
- Capability to choose the sex of unborn children
- Some control over weather or climate

The first twenty-five items on their list, however, were identified as ones which most people would see as "unambiguous examples of progress." These include:

- New sources of power for ground transportation (storage-battery, fuel-cell propulsion or support by electromagnetic fields, jet engine, turbine)
- Relatively effective appetite and weight control
- New and improved plants and animals
- New or improved uses of the oceans (mining, extraction of minerals, controlled "farming," source of energy)
- Multiple applications of lasers and masers for sensing, measuring, communicating, cutting, heating, welding, power transmission, illumination, destructive (defensive), and other purposes

Kahn and Weiner acknowledged that some people might question even these developments, but they dismissed this as a concern by arguing that most people would agree that these developments represent progress "at least for those who are in favor of progress" (Kahn and Weiner, 1967, pp. 710–713).

Here Kahn and Weiner illustrate one of the basic assumptions of the technocratic world view: that technological development is, for the most part, synonymous with progress. Those who question technological innovation and change, who critically evaluate the social and economic implications of such change, are by definition against progress (Kahn and Weiner, 1967; Kranzberg, 1980; Florman, 1980, 1981; Winner, 1977, 1986).

Science and technology are generally viewed as neutral from the technocratic perspective. They serve no particular interests but rather the general interests of all. Any problems which do arise with respect to technology are viewed as resulting from the uses to which technology is put rather than as being inherent within the technology itself. Pascarella argues, "We should constantly question the users of technology. Challenging its very existence is wrong, however, because the better life the whole world wants depends on appropriately used technology. The mysteries of our origin and our destiny compel us to continue learning and innovating" (1979, p. vii). Pascarella agrees with those who argue that the problems which we face come not from technology but from a failure of human beings to adapt to the technological world they have created. Furthermore, any negative effects which technology produces can and will be rectified by new and even more sophisticated technology. It is up to technology, then, to solve the problems which technology creates (Kahn and Weiner, 1967; Kranzberg, 1980; Florman, 1981).

Any debate which arises over technological issues (debate between corporate interests and environmental interests, for example) is viewed, at best, as debate among groups with competing good intentions and, at worst, as debate between those for progress and those against progress. Florman (1980, p. 28) argues that pesticides are good because they keep people from starving. But it is also good to oppose pesticides when they create havoc in the food chain. To drill for oil and transport it across the ocean is good. It is also good to prevent oil spills. Nuclear energy is good, and it is also good to try to eliminate radioactivity. These opposing activities are presented as sets of competing good intentions. The technocratic perspective provides little discussion of whether certain groups gain while others lose as a result of the decisions made with respect to technology. There is little discussion about economic or political power or about the role that power plays in shaping and directing technological development (Kranzberg, 1980; Florman, 1980, 1981).

Expertise is seen as necessary for decision making on technological issues due to the complexity of the issues involved. Technology supports social stratification by locating specialized knowledge in elite experts. As a result it becomes difficult for average citizens to play a role in decision making because of their lack of specialized knowledge. As such, human beings, rather than questions relating to technology, appear to pose the biggest problem from the technocratic perspective. There are many opinions as to how to handle the human problem, ranging from rapid social innovation (Kranzberg, 1980), to the elimination of political conflict (Fuller, 1969), to the development of a technology of human behavior (Skinner, 1971). Nonetheless, the emphasis from this perspective is on how human beings might adapt to technology rather than on developing technology compatible with the complexities of human life.

This applies to technology generally and to birthing technology specifically. Davis-Floyd (1992) gives numerous examples of how birth technology serves ritual purposes but not necessarily medical ones. As a result, the basic human needs and desires of birthing women are subordinated to the technology. One woman in Davis-Floyd's study (Diana Crosse) talks about her experience of being hooked to an external fetal heart monitor. She says, "As soon as I got hooked up to the monitor, all everyone did was stare at it. The nurses didn't even look at me anymore when they came into the room—they went straight to the monitor. I got the weirdest feeling that it was having the baby, not me" (Davis-Floyd, 1992, p. 107). Davis-Floyd points out that the circumstances of Diana's birth had been so completely defined by the technocratic model that even Diana began to feel that the machine was having the baby and she herself was relegated to the role of spectator.

While proponents of the technocratic world view argue that the complexity of technological issues requires that laypeople defer to experts for decision making regarding technology, many laypersons have demanded a voice in such decision making. Publications such as *Public Citizen* and *Consumer Reports* keep their readers aware of issues involving technology which touch all of us in our daily lives. Organizations such as the Center for Science in the Public Interest keep the public aware of a range of concerns about the quality of the food we eat, the air we breathe, and the water we drink. Citizens across the United States have become involved in efforts to document the effects of environmental hazards in their neighborhoods. One such person, Lois Gibbs, gained national recognition for the work that she and her neighbors did in her neighborhood near Love Canal, New York. When public officials turned their backs after citizens in the area complained that their many chronic illnesses and conditions were linked to chemicals which had been dumped in their neighborhood, Gibbs and her neighbors systematically documented the illnesses people were experiencing and insisted that officials take some action.

Appropriately, more decisions regarding technology are being made in the political process. As a result we have governmental bodies (such as the Consumer Product Safety Commission and the Environmental Protection Agency) for the purpose of protecting the public from technology for the sake of profit. While some of those who represent the technocratic perspective applaud public participation in the decision-making process, Kranzberg (1980) and Pascarella (1979) remind us that we cannot resolve our problems without technical experts. These experts are not viewed as representing particular interests, and decision making is not presented as a struggle between differing interests who wield different degrees of power and influence.

From this perspective, high technology is seen as a necessary precondition for just decision making. Many of our social problems remain because we have not yet developed the social innovations to accompany our technological innovations. Rather, our technological innovations have been used in the service of a society based upon competition and scarcity (Kranzberg, 1980).

POLITICAL-ECONOMIC CRITIQUES

The technocratic world view has been criticized by numerous authors including Ellul (1964), Schon (1971), Friedman (1973), Noble (1977),

Winner (1977, 1986), Alchon (1985), Rothman (1989), Wolin (1981), Dickson (1981, 1984), Broomfield (1980), and Morgall (1993). They argue that the technocratic perspective fails to look at the relationship among technology, politics, and the current state of international capitalism. An understanding of the relationship among these phenomena must underlie any analysis of technology in contemporary society.

Broomfield (1980, p. 29) argues that we need to recognize the "systematic relationship of high technology to the all-pervasive bureaucratic organization of our contemporary economic, political, and social structures." We cannot do away with big bureaucracy and keep high technology because they are systematically interrelated. Both Broomfield (1980) and Rothman (1989) remind us that when they talk about technology they are talking about more than just artifacts. They are also talking about the organization of their use. Rothman, specifically, talks about the ideology of technology as a way of thinking about the world in mechanical-industrial terms. This ideology influences the way we think about ourselves and about the world. The consistent themes of this ideology are order, productivity, rationality, and control. Rothman argues:

> In technological society we apply ideas about machines to people, asking them, too, to become more efficient, productive, rational, and controlled. We treat our bodies as machines, hooking them up to other machines, monitoring and managing bodily functions. When a doctor manages a woman's labor, controlling her body with drugs and even surgery it is to make her labor more efficient, predictable, rational. . . . When we think of parenting or raising our children, of our *relationships* with our children as a job to be done well, we are invoking the ideology of technology." (1989, p. 53)

Critics of the ideology of technology point out that it relies on the use of cost-benefit analysis as the basis for decision making. The basic principle underlying cost-benefit analysis is that it makes sense to prefer one alternative if its benefits in relation to costs are greater than they are for the next best alternative. In using cost-benefit analysis, numerical values are assigned to the costs and benefits involved. A price tag has to be put on all relevant concerns; otherwise, comparisons become impossible. The political implications of this method of decision making are obscured by claims that the technique is objective (Wolin, 1981). Dickson (1981) argues that cost-benefit analysis requires the oversimplification of complex phenomena and the use of subjective assessments (regarding, for example, the value of one's health, clean air, preservation of open spaces) in quantitative analysis.

Cost-benefit analysis fails to take into account values and issues which are not of interest to the corporate sector (Dickson, 1981). Health damage, for example, is measured in terms of lost earnings or lost productivity. While it is true that governmental agencies have been put in place to regulate the effects of technological development, Dickson (1981) points out that corporations have the ability to limit the influence of regulatory agencies, and in recognition of this, agencies mold their strategies into a form compatible with corporate interests.

The ground rules of liberal democracy are being replaced. Instead of a civic culture conducive to debating interests, values, and collective goals, there is a uniform discourse of calculation. According to Wolin (1981), the new public philosophy is one in which economics serves as the force for legitimating private-sector decision making and limiting public participation. Beliefs that economics serves as a neutral tool for decision making and that the system is one which responds to a broad spectrum of interests mask the importance of power relations. Economics, Wolin argues, acts as a public language which serves the needs of modern science, technology, capitalism, and the state. Dickson (1984) argues that the dominant political and economic forces not only determine the shape and uses of high technology but also control the production of scientific knowledge upon which such technology is based.

Rothman (1989) argues that in technological society ideas about machines are applied to people. We can see many examples of this in our everyday lives. In a recent infomercial advertising instructional videotapes for improving relationships between spouses, a couple spoke about the difficulties of marital communication. The man in the couple insisted that women are simply "wired differently" than men and that these tapes helped him to figure out what makes his wife tick. We evaluate people using the criteria developed for machines.

SCIENTIFIC OBJECTIVITY AS IDEOLOGY

Claims about the objectivity of science underlie claims about the value neutrality of technology. If it is the case that science is lacking in objectivity and neutrality, then technology must also be characterized by a lack of neutrality.

It is not unusual to hear many scientists and nonscientists alike make the distinction between the nature of inquiry which takes place in the realm of the social sciences and that which takes place in the natural sciences. Social science, it is assumed, is fraught with ambiguity because of the competing political and social values of those engaged in such inquiry. Natural (or "hard") science, by contrast, is often presumed to constitute an area of inquiry which is characterized by value neutrality and objectivity. As such, knowledge rooted in natural science is often thought to be invulnerable to the same kinds of analysis, interpretation, and criticism which are applied to knowledge rooted in other disciplines.

In recent years, however, a number of works have emerged which are critical not only of the uses to which natural science is put but also of the very nature of the scientific project. Science for these authors is not an objective, value-neutral pursuit of truth. While science does represent an effort to describe and explain reality, reality itself is a product of human thought and action (Bleier, 1984). Scholars have pointed out that science provides one way of knowing the world. Habermas (1971) has maintained that this kind of science is driven by our human interest in controlling physical, biological, and social environments. Strict science is conducted through the ever greater exercise of technical control over the conditions of physical, biological, and social behavior in order to determine outcomes and make precise predictions. If this kind of science is extended improperly into areas of human under-standing, emotion, and identity formation, it erodes human freedom and community. Nature is turned into an object to be manipulated through instruments rather than understood. The concept of nature as instrumentality precedes the development of all particular technical organization. This tech-nological a priori, however, is a political a priori in view of the fact that the transformation of nature involves the transformation of man and that man-made creations emanate from and return to a societal context.

Marcuse (1964) argues that to say that the evolution of scientific method merely "reflects" the transformation of natural into technical reality in the process of industrial civilization is to assume two separate realms: (1) science and scientific thought (with their internal concepts and their internal truth) and (2) the use and application of science in the social reality. The logical conclusion based on such an assumption is that the two realms do not determine each other, that pure science is not applied science but rather retains an identity apart from its utilization.

Observation and experiment, the methodological organization and coor-dination of data, propositions, and conclusions, Marcuse contends, never proceed in an unstructured, neutral space. They occur, rather, in a given universe of discourse and action. Science observes, calculates, and theorizes, he says, from a position in this universe. In this universe, technology provides the "rationalization for the unfreedom" (1964, p. 158) of many by making man's "unfreedom" appear neither as irrational nor as political but rather as the inevitable result of the technical apparatus which simultaneously increases life comforts and productivity. Technological rationality, therefore, enhances rather than threatens the legitimacy of domination. The scientific project, prior to any application and utilization, is tied to a specific societal project. Human emancipation, therefore, requires a new science.

In this regard Marcuse's argument parallels those made by Foucault (1977). Foucault maintains that scientific knowledge is part of the relations of power that define people for manipulation and control by such social institutions as medicine, criminal justice, and mental hospitals. Technical knowledge is part and parcel of institutions of control. It is part of an apparatus rather than a neutral objective account.

Feminist scholars present a critique of science which bears many similarities to these positions. In these arguments, however, gender does not emerge as a crucial category, while in feminist critiques of science, gender is the central category. Feminist scholars are critical of nonfeminist critiques of science because while such critiques do reject claims of scientific neutrality, they continue to support divisions between public and private, personal and impersonal, masculine and feminine. These divisions are implicit within the scientific project (Keller, 1985; Bleier, 1984; Fee, 1983; Harding, 1986). A feminist perspective identifies these divisions as central to the structure of modern science and society. We can see the world, Keller argues, divided into a multiplicity of dichotomies: public/private, masculine/feminine, objective/subjective, power/love. The masculine/feminine dichotomy serves to underlie the others, and the split between masculine and feminine needs to be understood not only as a relation of opposites but also as a dominant and subordinate relation (Bleier, 1984). A feminist perspective on science, then, leads us to ask questions which other critiques of science do not. Keller says, "It leads us to ask how ideologies of gender and science inform each other in their mutual construction, how that construction functions in our social arrangements, and how it affects men and women, science and nature" (1985, p. 8).

While there are certainly differences among feminists writing on gender and science issues, there are a number of basic points that constitute the core of the feminist argument. These points are succinctly presented by Fee (1983) in her arguments regarding scientific objectivity. If we accept the dominant liberal ideology of science, then the questions which emerge from a feminist perspective make no sense. Science is objective and value free. Scientific method is constructed to exclude potential sources of error from its final product, scientific knowledge. Man is a rational individual capable of creating rational knowledge of the world through a process of hypothesis testing, progressing toward a more complete understanding of nature. It is not the subjectivity of the scientist, then, that is seen as producing knowledge, but the objectivity of the scientific method. Subjectivity is viewed with suspicion as a possible contaminant of the process of knowledge production.

Fee points out, however, that there is a certain amount of ambiguity within the liberal tradition regarding the identity of rational "man." Liberal philosophy states that men are individuals capable of conceptualizing their self-interests and acting on them in a rational manner. Liberal feminism has adopted this tradition and has asked that women be included within the definition of man, with both men and women having the same rights and freedoms.

The liberal ideology of rational man, however, is actually dependent upon an unstated clause, that is, that the characteristics of "man" are actually the characteristics of males and that "rational man" is inextricably bound to his categorical opposite, "emotional woman." The construction of this political philosophy and views of human nature, then, depends upon a series of dualisms involving gender differences. If we begin with the masculine/feminine dichotomy, we can then identify a whole string of dichotomies that follow from this initial split. On the masculine side we can list rationality, objectivity, power, and public (or impersonal) life. The opposite categories can be found on the feminine side of the dichotomy: emotion, subjectivity, love (or nurturance), and private (or personal) life.

Fee argues that these ideas about male and female nature have long been part of Western philosophy, but by the mid-nineteenth century they were being formulated as an explicit part of scientific theory. Science was becoming the new source of authority, and gender differences could now be explained by scientific principles and natural law. There is, according to Fee, an important difference between science and religion and philosophy, which preceded science as sources of authority. Religion and philosophy, Fee argues, were never *intrinsically* male, although the female role in them was clearly limited and subordinate. The sciences, however, have been seen as masculine not only because the majority of scientists have historically been men but also because the very characteristics of science are perceived as sex linked. Masculine characteristics of rationality, objectivity, and emotional detachment are also the characteristics which are used to describe the scientific endeavor.

The belief in scientific objectivity can be used to mask a number of specific problems which a feminist critique of science identifies. The claim of scientific objectivity can be used to create distance between the production of scientific knowledge and the uses of that knowledge. Scientists, then, can be freed from any social or moral responsibility regarding the application of the knowledge they produce.

The notion of scientific objectivity can be understood as requiring a distance between scientific rationality and any emotional or social commitment. Rational thought is conceived as being clearly divorced from emotion, and emotion is certainly outside the realm of objectivity. Fee argues that the concept of scientific objectivity, when used to denote the separation of thought and feeling, may be used to devalue any positions expressed with emotional intensity. Feeling is suspect. The positions of those who are perceived as proceeding from rational thought are viewed as superior to the positions of those perceived as (or labeled as) proceeding from emotion. What emerges is yet another dualism between experts and laypersons where "experts" are perceived as representing rational thought and "laypersons" are thought to represent emotion combined with a lack of thought and information. Fee states:

> Everyone lacking scientific credentials can be made to feel uninformed, unintelligent, and lacking in the skills required for successful debate over matters of public policy. Those with sufficient wealth may be able to hire the scientific expertise needed to give their positions public validation, but those without wealth must bow to the superior knowledge of experts. Knowledge can, in this system, flow only in one direction: from expert to non-expert. There is no dialogue: the voice of scientific authority is like the male voice-over in commercials, a disembodied knowledge that cannot be questioned, whose author is inaccessible. (1983, pp. 18–19)

According to Fee and others (Bleier, 1984; Keller, 1985, Harding, 1986), science is characterized by a split between subject and object which legitimates the logic of the domination of nature. It is important, then, to view science as a part of human society determined by particular human aims and values and not as the depersonalized voice of abstract authority. We must be able to discuss the values and intentions of scientific knowledge, and we must not deny the social content of scientific knowledge. Fee argues that the production of scientific knowledge is highly organized and closely integrated with structures of political and economic power, and she points to several steps which must be taken in order to achieve a more fully human understanding of science. It is necessary to readmit the human subject into the production of scientific knowledge and accept science as a historically determined human activity. If we admit that scientific activity responds to specific social and political agendas, we can begin to see how science and scientists might relate in a different way to social and political questions.

Along these lines, Habermas (1971) has said that we have a human interest in developing knowledge that frees us from unnecessary social constraints and cultural definitions that block our capacities for self-development, responsibility, and participation in determining our lives. This "emancipatory" interest underlies critical science and the critique of ideology, including the misplaced use of science and technology for social and gender domination.

A feminist analysis of science (and, indeed, a feminist analysis generally) begins with a rejection of the split between public and private, objectivity and subjectivity, reason and feeling. From a feminist perspective, a dualistic mode is a cultural construction and the oppositions it poses are culture-bound concepts. Bleier states, "Hierarchies, relations of domination, subordination, power, and control are not necessarily inherent in nature but are an integral part of the conceptual framework of persons bred in a civilization constructed on principles of stratification, domination, subordination, power, and control, all made to appear natural" (1984, p. 200).

While the feminist critique of science is far reaching, feminist analysts do not reject all scientific claims as invalid nor do they deny all possibility of comprehending the world in rational terms. The success of any particular scientific endeavor, however, must be recognized as being limited by the context in which it arises (Keller, 1985). Feminist analysis, then, does not pose a choice between science as we know it and complete cultural relativism. Fee (1983) holds that the creation of knowledge through a constant process of practical interaction with nature, a willingness to consider all assumptions and methods as open to question, and the expectation that ideas will be critically evaluated are all aspects of scientific method which should be preserved.

There is some disagreement among feminist scholars as to whether or not a feminist science is possible. There are those (Harding, 1986) who argue that a feminist science is possible and preferable to what currently exists. Others are not so sure. Keller (1985), for example, argues that science as we know it developed only once in history. To talk about a "different" science, then, is to some extent a contradiction in terms. Still others argue that feminists are currently engaged in a critique of existing science and that there is no way within the present context to imagine another fully articulated scientific theory (Fee, 1983). We can, however, consider the criteria that a feminist science should fulfill. Fee states, "If we begin from the previous analysis we can say that a feminist science would not create artificial distinctions between the production and uses of knowledge, between thought and feeling, between subject and object, or between expert and non-expert. It would not be based on the divorce between subjectivity and objectivity, but would rather seek to integrate all aspects of human experience into our understanding of the natural world" (1983, p. 22).

Fee illustrates this position by using medical practice as an example. Medical practice, she argues, would be changed considerably if the subjective experience of the patient were thought to be a legitimate concern in medical practice and a necessary component of treatment or healing. A reevaluation of the importance of the patient's subjective experience has the effect of diminishing the overall authority of the physician. The women's health movement stands as an example of an organized effort aimed at insisting on a more reciprocal relationship between doctors and patients. By doing so, it has succeeded in gaining new visibility for women's experience and, Fee argues, this offers the potential for expanding the boundaries of scientific knowledge within medicine. This may, Fee says, require changes in our understanding of what is "real," change in the boundaries between the objective and the subjective, and more thoughtful inquiry into the relationship between mind and body. Such changes, however, mean neither the end of medical science nor a rejection of everything achieved by the earlier paradigm. Such changes do, however, offer the possibility of a more complete form of knowledge.

Fee's arguments regarding medical practice are directly relevant to the experiences of women in childbirth. Research demonstrates the ways in which the experiences of birthing women are marginalized and ignored (Rothman, 1989, 1982; Jordan, 1993; Martin, 1987; Oakley, 1984). Harrison (1982) argues that birthing women are often viewed as interfering in the relationship between the obstetrician and the fetus. The movement to create free-standing birth centers is due at least in part to this marginalization and objectification of birthing women.

SCIENCE, TECHNOLOGY, AND CHILDBIRTH

The logic of domination which characterizes science and the practice which informs it affects everyone. Nevertheless, it affects women in a particular way. In the case of medical practice, when women are the patients, the physician-patient relationship embodies the basic dualism between masculine and feminine. There is no shortage of evidence that women experience treatment by the medical profession which cannot be explained by the basic split between layperson and expert which characterizes medical practice in this society. Corea (1985a) argues that medical textbooks often express contemptuous attitudes toward women as well as inaccurate information and that medical students and faculty often harbor resentment toward women, both as medical students and as patients. Harrison (1982) documents numerous examples of mistreatment of female patients. In one instance Harrison recalls overhearing a conversation between an obstetrician-gynecologist with whom she was working and a fertility specialist:

Fertility specialist: I see you have a hysterectomy later today. Are you taking out the ovaries on her?

Ob-gyn: Well, I hadn't made up my mind yet, John. Why?

Fertility specialist: I'm looking for ovaries. I need some.

Ob-gyn: Well, I guess I could.

Fertility specialist: Don't do it for my sake. (1982, pp. 208–209)

Harrison cites examples not only of physical mistreatment, but also of verbal abuse which she witnessed as a resident in obstetrics and gynecology. She recalls a male colleague screaming at a birthing woman, "Push, push. You lazy female, push." Later this same man told Harrison, "Michelle, when people are in a subservient position, sometimes you just have to tell them what to do" (1982, pp. 198–199). Harrison argues that the presumption that women having babies are subservient to their doctors is implicit in obstetrics and that her own birth experience was no different. The hospital at which Harrison was in residence had a reputation for avoiding unnecessary intervention in childbirth and for its humane treatment of patients. Harrison demonstrates that, instead, women were frequently degraded, abused, and ignored.

The basic dualism which characterizes the physician-patient relationship for women is complicated when reproductive issues are involved. Once conception has been achieved it is only women who are directly involved in reproduction. Pregnant women stand as living symbols of the male/female dichotomy and as such seem to become particularly visible targets for mistreatment by physicians. Numerous authors have identified the extent to which pregnant women are characterized by physicians as being irresponsible, childlike, and incompetent to make decisions regarding their own well-being (Jordan, 1993; Rothman, 1989, 1982; Harrison, 1982; Arms, 1975; Ehrenreich and English, 1979). Incompetence on the part of pregnant women is made even more serious because it is not only their own health but the health of their fetuses which is at stake. The fetus provides another focus of attention for the physician. As mentioned before, many authors (Harrison, 1982; Rothman, 1982) argue that the dominant form of obstetrical practice is fetus-centered rather than woman-centered. This focus on the fetus encourages the use of invasive technology to gather information on the fetus. This technology, in turn, further erodes the autonomy of pregnant and birthing women by making them appear more and more superfluous to the birth process. Harrison argues that obstetricians might be more accurately termed pre-birth pediatricians or "feteotricians" (1982, p. 132).

The extent to which fetal rights and interests predominate over those of pregnant women is best illustrated through the example of postmortem maternal ventilation (PMV), a relatively low-tech procedure for keeping brain-dead women alive in order to sustain a pregnancy. Morgall argues:

The assessment of this procedure is an example of the predominant focus on fetal rights in the ethics debate today: standard, frequently used methods such as cost-effectiveness analysis were applied with the result that PMV was found to be cost-effective because it requires only standard hospital life-support equipment and decreases the need for high-cost prenatal technology. The procedure is therefore seen as the means of obtaining the goal (a life saved) at the lowest possible cost. A cost-effectiveness analysis does not question the ethics of making this procedure available or provide any criteria for its use. (1993, p. 193)

Hartouni (1991) draws attention to the discourse surrounding the practice of keeping brain-dead women alive to prolong a pregnancy. She asks her readers to consider a headline which appeared in the *San Francisco Chronicle* in July 1986 and read, "Brain Dead Mother Has Her Baby." The concept of motherhood as it is used here is a very particular one. Motherhood is equated with pregnancy and is reduced to a physiological function requiring no active participation. Certainly this concept of motherhood requires no conscious participation. Hartouni maintains that we need to consider an alternative concept which distinguishes between pregnancy and motherhood and which views motherhood as something which is socially constructed and historically specific (1991, pp. 30–31). Mothering is an activity, not an identity, and it is not necessarily gender specific (Ruddick, 1989; Rothman, 1989).

Jordan (1993) argues that high-technology birth contributes to the marginalization of birthing women. The degree of familiarity which women have with birth technology lessens as we move from low-tech artifacts to high-tech ones, and this has consequences for the experience of labor and birth. When a woman gives birth in a hammock or in her own bed, she has control over her experience. She can move around to facilitate her labor and to find positions which make her most comfortable (Jordan, 1993, p. 205). I found this to be true in my own research on women who give birth at home. They felt free to find positions which gave them comfort and support. They were able to move about freely and to find a rhythm to their labors. Because they were on their own territory, they felt uninhibited and empowered through the experience of birth. This type of birth experience does not happen in a hospital labor or delivery room where there is little opportunity for freedom of movement and little or no control on the part of birthing women.

Technologies also affect the nature of and the flow of information about birth. Jordan (1993, p. 209) argues that as we move from low technology to high technology a change occurs regarding who is in control of the information relevant to birth. In high-technology settings, control over the instruments and machinery which surround birth lies with the medical staff. The tools of birth are not touched by nonspecialists. Sometimes they cannot even be seen, as is the case with instruments covered by sterile cloths. The information which comes through high-tech machinery often requires expert interpretation so that it is inaccessible to birthing women themselves and it takes precedence over information from other sources. In hospitals it is the machinery that produces the knowledge upon which decisions are based.

In the high-tech birth environment there is what Jordan refers to as a bias toward upscaling. When a problem arises during the birth process, the solution to the problem is always sought at the next higher level of technology. It is rare for solutions to be sought at a lower level of technology. Jordan observes, "For example, if a woman's contractions slow down because she has been moved to a delivery table, she is not allowed to resume the previously effective position, but rather is given Pitocin to speed up labor, or perhaps a Cesarean" (1993, p. 212).

In the contemporary context, high technology has come to be equated with progressive medicine. In fact, high-technology birthing artifacts may have more symbolic value than use value (Jordan, 1993). It has been well documented, for example, that routine use of electronic fetal heart monitoring does not lead to improved outcomes (Jordan, 1993; Rothman, 1989; Ruzek, 1993; Arney, 1982). Yet the routine use of this technology is an accepted part of high-tech birth and is an important feature in the maintenance of the hierarchy of control.

Winner (1986) argues that we need to consider the ways in which technologies provide structure for human activity. Technologies are not merely tools but are also forces which reshape human activity and the meaning of that activity.

The technologies used throughout pregnancy and the birth process must be analyzed and understood as features of social relations and the exercise of power and control. They reflect the basic dualisms between the physician as expert and the birthing woman as layperson, and also between masculine and feminine. As Cockburn (1992, p. 42) argues:

Among the things gender may be able to clarify for us about technology is the nature of its implication in control, exploitation, and domination. For gender is not merely a relation of difference, it is one of asymmetry. Women commonly experience the masculine relations of technology as relations in which they are dominated and controlled. Some feel there is a connection between their own experience and what they observe to be the damaging relation of industrial technoscience with the natural environment.

Childbirth technologies serve to maintain the authority of the physician and to threaten the autonomy of birthing women. Women's reproductive experiences are defined and manipulated through the authority of technical language and procedures.

All of the technologies surrounding pregnancy and birth affect women in particularly intimate and important ways, but they also have important implications for society as a whole. At this point there are no effective societal mechanisms for decision making about and control over reproductive technologies. As these technologies become more invasive and involve greater and greater levels of surveillance and control (Oakley, 1984), such mechanisms become even more important (Morgall, 1993, pp. 189–190).

Morgall argues for a woman-specific assessment of new reproductive technology and identifies four reasons why this is important:

1. It is women's bodies which are the immediate objects of intervention.
2. Such technologies can affect changes in gender relations in society at large and within the family in particular.
3. Such technologies have an impact on concepts of maternity and paternity, and on social and cultural structures which shape women's lives.
4. Such technologies are key to genetic engineering.

Any adequate assessment of such technologies must include women's social and cultural experiences.

Davis-Floyd (1992) argues that medicine is a microcosm of American society in which the interests of science, technology, patriarchy, and institutions are viewed as superior to those of nature, individuals, families, and, most particularly, women. The hospital becomes the locus for the practice of technocratic medicine.

> The hospital is a highly sophisticated technocratic factory; the more technology the hospital has to offer, the better it is considered to be. As an institution, it constitutes a more significant social unit than the individual or the family, so the birth process should conform more to institutional than personal needs. As one physician put it, "There was a set, established routine for doing things and the laboring woman was someone you worked around rather than with." (Davis-Floyd, 1992, p. 55)

Birth creates a different set of problems within our technocratic culture, which rests on the assumption of man's superiority to nature. Birth is a process which can be neither predicted nor controlled. The dilemma in a technocratic culture becomes how to create a sense of cultural control over birth, which is a process resistant to such control. Another dilemma is how to get women to internalize the basic tenets of the technocratic model of reality, which amounts to asking women to "accept a belief system that inherently denigrates them" (Davis-Floyd, 1992, pp. 60–61).

The science of obstetrics mediates the cultural dilemmas which birth poses. It does so by (1) working out a philosophical rationale for the management of birth which interprets birth in terms of the technocratic mode and (2) by developing a set of ritual procedures which can be applied to the process of human reproduction to transform it into a process of human production, much like the production of any other technocratic artifact (Davis-Floyd, 1992, pp. 62).

An analysis of childbirth and the technologies which have come to define the medical model of birth serves to demonstrate the interrelationships among authority, technology, and gender. In the medical model, physicians and technicians not only have the power to define the birth process and to constrain the availability of options, but they also have appropriated the very experience of giving birth. The following chapter discusses the medical model and its implications for the experience of women in childbirth.

3

The Medical Model

Once there was a time when pregnant women quickened, and when this happened they knew they were with child. It might take place in the drawing room, as we know from the king's mistress, but most of the time it occurred while hoeing, cooking, or sewing. Making this known, the woman's declaration changed her state. A modern woman has not comparable power to redefine her social status by making a statement about her body. In our society, we are accepted as sick, healthy, or pregnant only when we are certified as such by a professional.

—Barbara Duden, *Disembodying Women*, p. 94

THE HOSPITAL, RISK, AND TECHNOLOGY

In our society it is difficult to think about birth in other than medical terms. The medical model shapes our basic assumptions about pregnancy and birth as well as the dominant practices surrounding these events. The beliefs and practices of the medical model are shaped by technocratic ideology. Davis-Floyd (1992) argues that it is the position of the medical profession that obstetrical procedures are determined by the physiological reality of labor and birth and, therefore, can be justified on "rational-technical" grounds. It has been demonstrated by a number of authors (Jordan, 1993; Davis-Floyd, 1992; Rothman, 1989; Martin, 1987; Oakley, 1984) that to fully understand the medical model of birth it is necessary to recognize that obstetric practice frequently has nothing to do with the "physiological reality" of labor and birth. Oakley comments on a photograph of a woman lying prone in order for her fetus to have its heart monitored:

It is, as one researcher has commented, most odd that, in view of the substantial evidence that the most unphysiologic thing one can do for either mother or baby is to lie mother flat on her back, it is a sobering thought that as we get more and more involved in . . . monitoring . . . the first thing we do is lie the mother on her back so we can drape all our recording gear on her and her baby. (1984, p. 183)

The power of the medical model to shape birth in the absence of evidence that medical procedures are scientifically warranted shows how technocratic ideology is institutionalized in practice. This chapter examines the assumptions and practices which underlie the medical model of birth and the ways in which the experiences of birthing women are shaped by this model.

Over 95 percent of all babies born in the United States are born in hospitals. When women are defined as patients in need of medical services, decision making shifts to doctors. Technical knowledge is viewed as the solid basis for decision making while the experiential knowledge of birthing women is discounted throughout pregnancy and, most particularly, during labor and birth within a hospital setting (Jordan, 1993; Eakins, 1986a; Rothman, 1989, 1982).

Preparation for birth is assumed to take place through formal channels including educational publications, childbirth classes, and physicians. A standard piece of advice contained in handouts from doctors to first-time mothers is to ignore the "old wive's tales," stories that they might hear from other women. Professional medical and technical information is seen as superior to the information which might be passed from woman to woman, from generation to generation (Jordan, 1993).

Access to prenatal care and childbirth preparation is dramatically influenced by race as well as by class. As one might expect, well-educated middle- and upper-class women have the greatest access to prenatal care and are most likely to take childbirth education classes. It is estimated that one out of every three pregnant women (about 3 million women every year) receives inadequate prenatal care. Among black women in the United States in 1988, only 61 percent received prenatal care from a biomedically trained practitioner. In the same year, 58 percent of Native American and Mexican American women received such care. The figure for Puerto Rican women and Central and South American women was 63 percent (Jordan, 1993, p. 57). At the same time that Jordan cites these statistics, however, she also points to the importance of carefully considering what actually leads to better birth outcomes. While it is widely believed that biomedical prenatal care is necessary for a healthy pregnancy, it is not clear what aspects of biomedical care are most directly related to healthy pregnancy and birth. Those things which have been demonstrated to correlate positively with birth outcome are higher income, higher education, and better nutrition. These factors also correlate with an inclination to seek prenatal care (Jordan, 1993, p. 57).

Once a woman enters a hospital to give birth, she is likely to be subjected to an array of high-technology devices and procedures. Usually an intravenous drip will be started. This provides some necessary calories since food intake is usually restricted. It also serves as preparation for administering Pitocin (a drug used to induce labor or to speed up labor) and some painkilling medications later in the labor.

Most labors in the United States are monitored with electronic fetal monitors, either an external one or the more invasive internal type. Laboring women usually receive some type of anesthetic or analgesic for pain relief. Labors are often induced or sped up with Pitocin. Jordan (1993) maintains that 80 percent of women birthing in hospitals in the United States have their labors augmented with Pitocin. Other common practices include artificial rupturing of the amniotic sac to speed up labor and the routine use of episiotomy, a cut in the perineal tissue to enlarge the vaginal opening (Harrison, 1982; Rothman, 1982; Stewart and Stewart, 1976). Cesarean sections are also a common occurrence in U.S. hospitals. The current rate of Cesarean sections in the United States is 22.7 percent (Ruzek, 1993).

Underlying these practices is the view of the body as a "machine" and the doctor as a "mechanic" (Harrison, 1982; Rothman, 1982). Rothman discusses the way in which doctors are taught to use a variety of drugs and procedures to facilitate "normal delivery":

> Once the body is conceptualized as a machine, then it is going to be treated in much the same way as any other machine in our society—pushed to be more efficient, more economic, faster, neater, and quieter. An infinite number of procedures and interventions are so readily normalized because that fits in with our view of the world: one is compelled to take action in order to get results. (1982, p. 40)

Emily Martin (1987) looks at how the obstetrical literature views labor. The uterus is viewed as an involuntary muscle; it, rather than the birthing woman, actually does the work. The uterus is judged as to whether it produces efficient or inefficient contractions, and whether a labor is good or poor is a feature of how much progress is made within a particular period of time. According to Martin:

> A woman's labor, like factory labor, is subdivided into many stages and substages. The first stage includes the latent phase (slow effacement and

dilation of the cervix to 3 or 4 cm); the active phase is further subdivided into the phase of acceleration, the phase of maximum slope and the phase of deceleration. The second stage includes the descent of the baby down the birth canal and its birth; and the third stage includes the separation and delivery of the placenta. (1987, p. 59)

Not only is labor divided into stages and substages, but every stage is also expected to progress at a particular rate. Failure to progress at these rates leads to a diagnosis of several "disorders" associated with labor.

Where does the laboring woman fit into this picture? On the one hand, since uterine contractions are assumed to be involuntary, women are of little importance in the process, particularly during dilation and prior to pushing. Yet women are constantly being evaluated during labor. They are told whether they are doing well or not and how much time remains in each stage. Women are viewed as "laborers" needing to be managed. Martin argues that what emerges are two juxtaposed images. On the one hand, there is the image of the uterus as the machine that produces the baby; on the other hand, there is the image of the woman as laborer who produces the baby. Sometimes the two come together—the woman laborer whose uterus machine produces the baby (Martin, 1987, p. 63). Harrison relates the notations that she made on a patient's chart as a resident in obstetrics and gynecology: "NSD (normal spontaneous delivery) from ROA (right occiput anterior) over ML Epis. (midline episiotomy) of male infant, Apgar 9/10. EBL (estimated blood loss) 50 cc., repair 3–0 chromic sutures. Mother to RR (recovery room) good condition. Infant to nursery" (1982, p. 84). This, Harrison reports, is the standard way of describing the more common vaginal birth within a hospital setting. This way of describing birth in technical, mechanical terms reflects the view of the body as a machine and the woman as marginal laborer.

The practice of hospitalizing women for childbirth is relatively recent. In 1900, 50 percent of births in the United States were home births attended by midwives. By 1930, 15 percent of births in the United States were attended by midwives, 80 percent of whom lived in the South (Leavitt, 1986). Over the course of the twentieth century, childbirth has become increasingly medicalized. In 1920, Dr. Joseph DeLee presented a paper entitled "The Prophylactic Forceps Operation" before the American Medical Association. In the paper he argued that birth was a horrifying experience for both mother and baby requiring the aid of surgical intervention. For the infant, he argued, birth was similar to having one's head squeezed in a slowly closing door. DeLee's remedy was to sedate laboring women and to make an incision of several inches to enlarge the vaginal opening so that the fetus could be removed with forceps (Arney, 1982; Edwards and Waldorf, 1984; Rothman, 1982). In DeLee's words:

> Labor has been called, and still is believed by many to be, a normal function. It always strikes physicians as well as laymen as bizarre, to call labor an abnormal function, a disease, and yet it is a decidedly pathological process. Everything, of course, depends on what we define as normal. If a woman falls on a pitchfork, and drives the handle through her perineum, we call that pathologic—abnormal, but, if a large baby is driven through the pelvic floor, we say that is natural, and therefore normal. If a baby were to have its head caught in a door very lightly, but enough to cause cerebral hemorrhage, we would say it is decidedly pathologic, but when a baby's head is crushed against a tight pelvic floor, and a hemorrhage in the brain kills it, we call this normal, at least we say that the function is natural, not pathologic. (Quoted in Arney, 1982, pp. 54–55)

DeLee saw labor as a pathologic process. He believed that few women escaped damage from labor and that many babies were killed or damaged as a result of labor and birth. He justified his recommendations on the grounds that they prevented the tearing of the perineum (pelvic floor), as well as more serious consequences for birthing women such as prolapsed uteri and tears in the vaginal wall. His proposed procedures could also prevent brain damage in newborns. By the 1930s DeLee's recommendations had become standard practice in many hospitals (Wertz and Wertz, 1977).

Despite a great deal of acceptance of the routine use of episiotomy and forceps advocated by DeLee, the definition of childbirth as pathological was not without problems. Contradictions surrounding this issue can be found even in DeLee's own writings. Childbirth was pathological and, then again, it was not. In order to resolve this contradiction, obstetrics introduced the notion of what Arney calls "pathological potential." While birth was essentially normal and natural, the chance for something to go wrong was always present (Arney, 1982, p. 54). This constant threat of danger meant that births could not be separated into the "normal" and the "abnormal." Rather, all births had the potential to become abnormal. It was important, then, that births be attended by those trained to recognize the signs of pathology, obstetricians themselves.

Central to the view which sees all births as potentially pathological is the idea of risk. Over the years obstetricians have tried to develop systems of predicting which women are at risk for developing complications (Oakley and Houd, 1990). Underlying the risk approach are several assumptions about birth. This approach views the "delivery" as the most important aspect of maternal health and maternity care. Obstetricians become advocates for the fetus and the newborn while the birthing woman becomes a passive object. The separation of the mother and the fetus is characteristic of the medical model of birth. The risk approach assumes not only that the mother and the fetus are separate, but also that they are at odds. There is a distrust of the mother as the best and most obvious advocate for the fetus. Mothers are frequently portrayed as being unable to make the best decisions for themselves and their children regarding pregnancy and birth. The fetus is portrayed as being held captive by a mother who does not have the best interests of the fetus at heart.

While separation of the mother and fetus is now characteristic of the medical model, the isolation of the fetus from the mother is a relatively recent conceptual development. Arney (1982) argues that around 1940, the field of obstetrics began to characterize the fetus as a separate entity. The 1941 edition of *Williams Obstetrics* uses the term "fetal distress" for the first time in its text. By 1976, *Williams Obstetrics* had added a new chapter on fetal health, and more recently obstetrician-gynecologists have moved toward practicing "maternal-fetal" medicine (Ruzek, 1993).

While new technologies certainly helped to make the mother/fetus separation possible, this new focus on the fetus gave obstetricians a new weapon against women who were becoming critical of the way obstetrics treated women. Obstetrical interventions no longer had to focus on the mother but could focus on the fetus instead. As Arney points out, "Obstetricians became fetal advocates and women were left to mount their struggle against an adversary who had acquired a potent ally in the fetus" (Arney, 1982, p. 137).

The maternal/fetal dichotomy has led to a legal struggle over the rights of the mother versus those of the fetus. In October 1986 charges of fetal abuse were brought against Pamela Rae Stewart. She was charged with causing the death of her son by disobeying her doctor's orders regarding her placenta previa, a condition in which the placenta partially or completely covers the cervical opening. Stewart was accused of being in violation of Section 270 of the California Penal Code, which requires parents to provide clothing, food, shelter, and medical care for their children (Ashford, 1986–87, p. 7). Lawyer Margery Shaw argues, "Once a pregnant woman has abandoned her right to an abortion and has decided to carry her fetus to term, she incurs a 'conditional prospective liability' for negligent acts toward her fetus if it should be born alive" (Arditti, Klein, and Minden, 1984, p. 345). According to this view, courts and legislatures should take all available steps to insure that fetuses who are carried to term are not handicapped by the negligence of others.

This issue of maternal/fetal separation has come to a head around the issue of court-ordered Cesarean sections (Rothman, 1989). When women in late pregnancy or in labor have disagreed with their physicians over decisions regarding the pregnancy or labor, doctors have asked the courts to intervene. In a number of cases, courts have issued orders forcing women to undergo Cesarean sections in the name of fetal protection (Gallagher, 1984).

The concept of the fetus as separate from the mother has become part of our popular cultural understanding. It is common for people to speak of the "unborn child" and to think of the fetus as a separate being, rather than as part of its mother's body. Pregnant women are warned about their responsibility to avoid drugs and alcohol. They are admonished to eat well and to engage in healthy living. The tone of this advice is threatening rather than benevolent. Pregnant women are portrayed as the enemies of their own fetuses.

Forced Cesarean sections, maternal liability for defects in their offspring, and charges of fetal abuse are all aspects of a trend which pits fetal rights against maternal rights. Fetuses and mothers are viewed as separate entities, and doctors' orders are sometimes given the force of law. The maternal/fetal dichotomy, however, is a false one. Since the fetus is part of the mother's body, nothing can be done to it without also doing something to the mother. Gallagher argues that forcing women by court order to undergo medical treatment for which they have not given informed consent violates the well-established legal principle that "bodily integrity is basic to human dignity and self-determination" (Gallagher, 1984, p. 65). These efforts represent the ultimate attempt on the part of the medical establishment (supported by legal precedent) to control the behavior of women during pregnancy, labor, and birth (Gallagher, 1984; Harrison, 1982; *Women's Rights Law Reporter*, 1982).

All births are viewed as potentially life threatening, particularly for the fetus. As a result, birth is seen as requiring surveillance and control to monitor any deviation from what is judged to be normal. The tools of surveillance are many. They include a host of technical procedures, screening and diagnostic tests, and monitoring devices. Some of these are used during pregnancy, including ultrasound screening, alpha-fetoprotein testing, chorionic villus sampling, and amniocentesis. Others, such as electronic fetal monitoring, drugs to induce or speed up labor, and Cesarean section, are used during labor and birth. The risks involved with the routine use of such procedures, rates of diagnostic errors, and the benefits of other low-tech alternatives are rarely discussed.

Ruzek (1993) argues that advice to pregnant and birthing women often lacks information about the actual incidence of negative outcomes of procedures within a particular population. In the case of electronic fetal monitoring, for example, women often are not told that the conditions which might be "prevented" through the use of the monitor are extremely rare. Despite a lack of evidence about the benefits of electronic fetal monitoring, this remains a routine part of labor in many hospitals. There is very little consideration of risk relative to benefits for high-technology procedures. Rather, high-technology is viewed as the solution to the problems of poor birth outcomes. When low-technology approaches, including prenatal care, smoking cessation, and nutrition supplementation, are considered, they are held to much higher standards of efficacy and cost-effectiveness. As Ruzek states, what is actually being compared here are capital-intensive versus labor-intensive technologies:

> The cutting-edge interventions involve the development and sale of machines—machines that are profitable to produce and market worldwide. Many of these machines are marketed as a way to avoid labor costs. EFM [electronic fetal monitoring], for example, is often touted as an alternative to having more labor nurses. The labor-intensive, low-technology interventions are viewed as too costly, not because they are not cost-effective. They are costly because they do not generate profit and without the promise of profit, they are not aggressively marketed. Thus, the entire medical-scientific literature is biased in the direction of assessing capital-intensive products over labor-intensive approaches to reducing birth risks. (1993, p. 401)

The risk approach has been criticized for a variety of reasons. Oakley and Houd (1990) argue against its methodology. The risk approach is scientifically awkward because in order to identify deviations from normal, it is first necessary to define what is normal. Obstetricians are inadequate in their knowledge of the many variations within normal birth. Normality is an artifact of medical procedures, settings, and discourses. Consequently, birth can be defined as normal only in retrospect.

Moreover, the belief that birth is life threatening instills fear in women. This fear leads to a greater dependence upon the medical model of birth and upon medical practitioners, which promise the "safest" route through this risky process. Birth within a high-technology hospital, with a physician in attendance, becomes the only way to contain the risk.

The hospital setting is very important because it is the core location of medical procedures and knowledge. It controls what can be seen and by doing so maintains the medical model. As Rothman points out, "The institutions of medicine prevent anomalies in the model from showing up. This is done most effectively . . . by defining all anomalies as pathological, and treating them" (1982, p. 284). The hospital setting institutionalizes the social relationships, power differences, knowledge, and our beliefs about birth. These beliefs bolster the practice of birthing in hospitals through the medical model.

Just as the hospital supports the medical model, it undermines birthing women. Within the high-technology hospital, what women know through their bodily experience is either given no status or is interpreted in terms of the medical model. Physicians in the same setting are recognized as having "authoritative knowledge." Authoritative knowledge is not necessarily correct, but is, rather, the knowledge which all of the participants agree counts within a particular situation. It is the knowledge which is seen as the legitimate basis for making decisions and for justifying actions taken. There is no room for competing information:

> What the woman knows and displays by virtue of her bodily experience has no status. Within the official scheme of things, she has nothing to say that matters in the actual management of her birth. Worse, her knowledge is nothing but a problem for her and the staff. What she knows emerges not as a contribution to the store of data relevant for decision-making, but rather as something to be cognitively suppressed and behaviorally managed. In the labor room authoritative knowledge is privileged, the prerogative of the physician, without whose official certification of the woman's state, the birth cannot proceed. (Jordan, 1993, p. 157)

Having authoritative knowledge gives the physician the power to make judgments and pronouncements about the events surrounding birth. It is the physician, for example, who gives official permission for the birthing woman to begin pushing her baby out. The time of the physician's pronouncement is marked and this time becomes the official beginning of the second stage of labor. This official record, however, does not necessarily match the birthing woman's experience. She may have felt the urge to push prior to the physician's arrival and, if left to her own devices, might indeed have started to push earlier.

In observing birth in U.S. hospitals, Jordan (1993) witnessed many examples of the artificial and arbitrary identification of the stages of labor. She argues that these arbitrary time frames become part of the official statistics regarding average lengths of labors and then are put to normative use in managing labor in hospital settings. This stands as a direct example of Rothman's point that the setting of birth helps to control what can be seen and consequently helps to control what is known about birth.

The setting is also directly related to the level of birthing technology used. The routine use of high-technology equipment in a hospital setting contributes to the marginalization of birthing women. They lack access to the information provided by hospital technology, which often requires expert interpretation. Often women themselves begin to believe that the machines know more about how their labor is going than they do.

SCIENTIFIC RATIONALE

The rationale for the medical model is that it is both scientific and effective in a way that other models for birth are not. It is often the case, however, that the practices and procedures supported by the medical model are neither scientific nor effective (Oakley and Houd, 1990; Jordan, 1993; Arney, 1982; Rothman, 1989, 1982).

Most hospital births in the United States involve some type of medication for pain relief. Rothman argues, however, that the pain which birthing women experience does not correspond to the medical expectations regarding pain in childbirth. Women who have experienced unmedicated births usually report that the first stage of labor, cervical dilation, is the most painful part of labor. The second stage, pushing and the birth itself, is reported to be less painful. According to the medical model, though, it is the second stage which is thought to be most painful and which is treated with the most potent pain medication (Rothman, 1982, pp. 82–83).

The anesthetic of choice for many women is epidural anesthesia. An epidural involves injecting a local anesthetic between the vertebrae of the lower back, into the epidural space of the spinal column. In many hospitals over 80 percent of birthing women receive epidurals (Jordan, 1993). Because epidurals can free women from pain without dulling the mental faculties, they are commonly used during Cesarean sections so that women can remain conscious throughout the surgery. They can also be used in lower doses during vaginal birth for complete or nearly complete pain relief. Jordan (1993) reports that when epidurals are given effectively they can eliminate pain while reducing neither the urge nor the ability to push. Applied less skillfully, an epidural can deaden sensations, reducing the ability to push and increasing the likelihood of a forceps delivery or a Cesarean section. There is a great deal of variation in how individual women will respond to an epidural. Some women will still experience pain, while others will feel nothing and be unable to push. If the medication is given too early in labor, it can slow the labor down. The risks of epidurals to mothers include the increased likelihood of forceps deliveries and of Cesarean sections, hypotension (lowered blood pressure), and central nervous system depression. The risks to babies include oxygen deprivation, slowing of the heart rate, and an increase in the acidity of the blood (Jordan, 1993; Ashford, 1985; Harrison, 1982; Kelly, 1979; Gilgoff, 1978).

Many drugs which are given for pain relief have the effect of slowing down labor. Artificial stimulation of labor then becomes necessary. As mentioned earlier, the drug used to induce or stimulate labor is Pitocin. A number of risks have been associated with Pitocin. The effects of this drug are often unpredictable. In some women there is little effect, while in other women labor intensifies dramatically. In laboring women, Pitocin can cause uterine spasms resulting in premature separation of the placenta, laceration of the birth canal, and possible uterine rupture. Pitocin can also lead to fetal distress due to a lack of oxygen and to intracranial hemorrhage. Pitocin has also been linked to an increase in neonatal respiratory problems (Jordan, 1993, p. 77; Edwards and Waldorf, 1984, p. 209).

Electronic fetal monitoring during labor is used routinely in many hospitals, despite any clear evidence of its effectiveness. When an external monitor is used, a laboring woman has a belt strapped around her abdomen. On the belt are a set of sensors which send signals to the monitor. The sensors measure the fetal heart rate and the strength of uterine contractions. If an internal monitor is used, the fetal heart rate is recorded by an electrode which is attached to the fetal scalp. If the amniotic sac is still intact, it will have to be broken in order for the internal monitor to be used. An information sheet on fetal heart monitoring made available by Corometrics Medical Systems and given out at some hospitals offers consolation to women who are concerned about attaching electrodes to the scalps of their fetuses. "The application of the spiral electrode will make one tiny needle mark on the baby's skin which will disappear usually in approximately 2 or 3 days." The electrode is attached to lead wires. Once the electrode is in place the lead wires are attached to a small leg plate on the mother's upper thigh. The wires extend from the leg plate to the monitor. Monitoring can also be accomplished by telemetry, a process which allows information to be transmitted from one location to another. The transmitter is attached to the mother's abdomen by an elastic strap. It collects information on fetal heart rate and maternal contractions from either an external transducer or an internal catheter and the spiral electrode. The transmitter can relay information to a receiver connected to the fetal monitor. Telemetry eliminates the need for the mother to be connected directly to the fetal monitor, allowing her some mobility within a limited area of the hospital.

Oakley (1984) argues that regardless of whether monitoring devices actually require physical passivity on the part of the laboring woman, they imply it ideologically. What monitoring and other forms of obstetric technology make possible is the gathering of information about the fetus without the active participation of the laboring woman. In Oakley's words, "As the 'iron curtain' of the mother has been swept aside revealing the womb and its contents in their full glory, it has become no longer necessary to consult mothers about their attitudes" (1984, p. 183).

Martin (1987) argues that with the standard monitors doctors, nurses, and technicians look at the monitor's printout to determine what is going on with the labor. They do not look at the laboring woman, and it is becoming more difficult for women to avoid the technology available in hospitals. Taking long walks around the hospital to avoid being hooked up to the monitor is ineffective when monitoring can be accomplished through telemetry.

Fetal monitors were originally used to monitor high-risk births but soon became routine for low-risk births as well. Ruzek (1993) points out that because monitors were marketed prior to 1976, when the Food and Drug Administration was mandated to regulate medical devices, the monitors did not undergo the same kinds of stringent premarket application procedures which are now in place. While the benefits of monitoring have been highly touted in the medical literature, a number of authors point out that evidence on fetal monitoring is ambiguous at best. Banta and Thacker (1979) argue that a careful review of the literature indicates little increased benefit from electronic fetal monitoring when compared with auscultation (listening with a stethoscope). Haverkamp et al. (1976) compared two groups of high-risk laboring women. One group was electronically monitored while the other was monitored by nurse auscultation. Perinatal outcomes were similar in the two groups but Cesarean section rates were 2.5 times higher in the electronically monitored group. While this study has been criticized for bias in the sample of women studied (Arney, 1982), a second study published by Haverkamp et al. (1979) confirmed their earlier findings. Shy et al. (1990) found that among premature children the incidence of cerebral palsy was higher in children whose births had been electronically monitored as compared with a group monitored through auscultation. Rothman (1982) argues that electronic fetal monitoring is both expensive and dangerous. Even for those women and babies who do not have their health compromised, fetal monitoring has a significant impact on the quality of the birth experience. Despite a lack of evidence of the benefits of routine monitoring, it remains a standard part of labor in most hospitals.

Cesarean sections carry other negative consequences beyond the physical risks and discomfort. Martin (1987) interviewed women about their birth experiences. She describes the feelings of alienation and violation which women felt following Cesarean birth. The following are quotes from some of the women interviewed by Martin:

I felt as if I were being crucified—both arms stretched out and pinned down spread eagle.

It was like a feeling of rape, completely out of control. My body was totally violated. I felt nobody cared. You wear cheap clothes and a lot of make-up and if you're raped, it's your fault. I felt the same thing with the Cesarean.

I had difficulty believing that I had, in fact, borne my seven-pound, six-ounce daughter. At times during those first few postpartum days, she seemed more like a doll handed to me by my obstetrician. (1987, pp. 84–85)

These women clearly saw themselves as passive objects, having something done to them rather than actively doing something on their own. They felt isolated, alienated, and violated. Yet some physicians have expressed an inability to understand why women so much prefer delivery "from below" to delivery "from above" (Rothman, 1982, p. 181).

Recent research compares Cesarean section rates with rates of vaginal birth after Cesarean (VBAC) among four categories of hospitals. Federal government hospitals have the lowest Cesarean rates (17 percent). State and local government hospitals have a 21.1 percent Cesarean rate. The Cesarean rate at not-for-profit hospitals is 22.4 percent. The highest rates of Cesarean sections are in for-profit hospitals (25.3 percent). A similar pattern can be observed if VBAC rates are examined. Federal hospitals have a VBAC rate of 32.6 percent. Not-for-profit hospitals have a rate of 23.7 percent. State and local government hospitals have a rate of 23.2 percent. The lowest VBAC rates (16 percent) are found in for-profit hospitals (Public Citizen Health Research Group, 1994).

Information which links rates of Cesarean sections to the types of insurance which women have and to the types of hospitals in which women give birth raises serious questions about why many Cesarean sections are carried out. There is little disagreement over the argument that current Cesarean rates are too high. Yet physicians continue to justify individual Cesarean sections as necessary. Martin (1987) argues that it is significant that Cesarean section requires the most management by physicians and is seen as providing the best products. There is a belief that Cesarean birth leads to perfect babies, an apparent legacy of the idea that labor and vaginal birth are intrinsically traumatic to the baby. There is no doubt that Cesarean sections give greater power and control to physicians in relation to laboring women. Cesarean sections are also consistent with the technocratic view of the body as a machine which can be tinkered with and fixed. Widespread acceptance of technocratic values and a belief in the medical model lead the public to accept extraordinarily high Cesarean section rates in the face of strong evidence that many sections are unnecessary and are being done (or not done) for economic gain.

Researchers estimate that a Cesarean rate of 12 to 15 percent would save over $1 billion per year in physician fees and hospital charges. The money that is now being wasted on unnecessary Cesarean sections could be spent on preventing low birthweight in babies and caring for children and adults whose health care needs currently go unmet (Public Citizen Health Research Group, 1994).

Recent research suggests that having a supportive person with a birthing woman throughout labor can significantly reduce the rate of intervention including the rate of Cesarean section. In a study conducted by Kennell et al. (Jordan, 1993, p. 66), 402 healthy first-time mothers, all in active labor, were randomly assigned to one of two groups—supported or observed—upon arrival at the hospital. Both groups were compared with a control group. Those in the supported group were accompanied by a "doula" during labor and birth. A doula is a woman who provides comfort and support by talking to the laboring woman, holding her hand, rubbing her back, and offering encouragement. She might be a layperson, or she might have special training or experience. The supported group had a Cesarean section rate of 8.1 percent compared with 13.0 in the observed group and 18.1 in the control group.

For a number of years many researchers have argued that catecholamines (stress hormones including adrenaline and noradrenaline) produced by the fetus during labor are actually harmful to the fetus and that mothers should accept anesthesia in order to lessen their effects. Other evidence indicates, however, that this is not the case. Lagercrantz and Slotkin (1986) argue that catecholamines actually help the fetus by offering protection from hypoxia and by enhancing the ability of the fetus to adapt after birth. These researchers note that catecholamine levels positively correlate with higher Apgar scores in babies who are moderately asphyxiated, indicating that the hormones help to counteract the effects of oxygen deprivation. They also suggest that babies delivered by elective Cesarean section prior to the onset of labor miss the benefits of the surge of these hormones which occurs during labor.

Jordan (1993) maintains that physicians know that the best thing you can do during a normal birth is nothing, but that their professional training and the circumstances of their work make it almost impossible for them to do nothing during labor and birth. Part of the anxiousness about "doing something" has to do with the social awkwardness of a group of people standing around with nothing to do. Jordan argues:

> Interestingly, it is not speed but activity that emerges as the motivating force in these situations. As long as everybody is doing the things they

are trained to do, socially awkward situations do not arise. An episiotomy (an incision to enlarge the vaginal opening), for example, will get the baby born a few minutes faster, but the physician may spend half an hour or more sewing it up afterwards; so there is no saving in time. The interactional advantage is that this half hour is filled with appropriate activity for the delivery team rather than with inactive and awkward silence. (1993, pp. 61–62)

THE EXPERIENCES OF BIRTHING WOMEN

In the course of over ten years of research on childbirth, I have conducted interviews with women who have had both hospital and home birth experiences. The descriptions of the hospital experiences among the women I interviewed reflect the characteristic features of the medical model. The women describe themselves in unfamiliar settings where they exercised no control. They felt they should not make too much noise, should do what they were told, and should be as cooperative as possible.

None of the women I interviewed was satisfied with her hospital experience, but the reasons for this dissatisfaction were different. One woman, whom I will call Julia, said that initially she felt that her hospital experience had been fine. She had an episiotomy but otherwise there was little intervention. Two weeks following her birth, however, Julia suffered a hemorrhage. Her doctor was unable to explain why this had happened. Julia found this very upsetting because she was afraid it would happen following any subsequent births. In addition, Julia found her doctor's attitude to be very patronizing. He said that she should not worry about the cause of the hemorrhage, that everything would be okay.

Susan had planned a home birth but ended up in the hospital with a Cesarean section. Her baby was in a breech position, but she felt her doctor was much too anxious to intervene. In Susan's opinion, the Cesarean was unnecessary. She was disappointed in the way the birth turned out. She had been in labor for over ten hours before the doctor suspected that the baby was in a breech position. She felt that if more time had been taken, she could have birthed her baby and surgery could have been avoided.

Lynn had planned a hospital birth but had very clear ideas about what she wanted her birth to be like. She wanted as little intervention as possible and searched until she found a doctor who was willing to agree to her wishes. She put them in writing and had her doctor sign the list as an indication that he had agreed to her requests. Lynn describes the early part of her labor as wonderful. She was at home with her husband. They had a whirlpool bath which she used for relaxation. She describes feeling the progress of labor and moving around and changing positions in response to her contractions. Everything changed once she arrived at the hospital.

Lynn describes the nurses on duty as being annoyed at circumstances in general and at her in particular. She arrived at the hospital just prior to giving birth, and the nurses proceeded to scream at her through the rest of her labor and birth. Although Lynn had made very specific arrangements with her doctor beforehand, he was not on call and was not present at the birth. In fact, no doctor was present for the birth. Both Lynn and her husband were willing to question the judgment of the nurses; still, they found the nurses to be threatening and intimidating.

A doctor did show up about one and a half hours after the birth. What follows is Lynn's account of what happened:

> But after I had the baby another doctor did come. It was six o'clock on Sunday morning. He was drunk. He had obviously been up all night drinking. There was a mirror at the bottom of the delivery table. I could see him taking his bare hands and he literally tore me apart with his bare hands. I could see. I could obviously feel. He was drunk. It was not a good experience. And then he proceeded to sew me up without any anesthesia. I could see blood squirting out as he ripped me apart with his bare hands. He was drunk. All the while he was talking about how he wanted to get a sandwich from 7-Eleven. I was laid on this table, my legs were up in stirrups. I was saying stop, that hurts. I started screaming. I was in pain. It hurt.

Lynn had entered pregnancy with the confidence that birth will, in most instances, happen on its own if interference does not occur. She had consciously chosen a practitioner who shared her views and who expressed a willingness to respect her wishes. Despite her best efforts, she had a hospital experience during which she was intimidated and violated.

Pat had planned to give birth at a free-standing birth center. The dates of her pregnancy had been miscalculated. When she went into labor a month prior to the calculated due date, the nurse-midwives at the birth center believed that Pat was going to have a premature baby. They estimated the baby's weight to be less than five pounds. Under these circumstances, Pat was transferred to a hospital. She was given Pitocin to stimulate her labor. In her words, "There was a lot of interference with the birth." It turned out that the baby was not premature. He weighed six and a half pounds at birth, and in Pat's opinion, the "interference" had been unnecessary.

The specific circumstances of each of these births were different. In each instance, however, the birthing woman felt that she did not have control over the birth. The women felt that hospital procedures were unnecessary intrusions into the birth process and none of the women mentioned here returned to the hospital for subsequent births. Women who wish to avoid unnecessary intrusions often find it difficult if not impossible within the hospital setting. Often the requests are ignored and the women making them are viewed with contempt. During the course of my research I had a discussion with a top administrator at a large medical center about the desire of women to avoid episiotomy, a cut in the perineum made just prior to birth to enlarge the vaginal opening. He seemed to have some difficulty understanding why women would want to avoid this and responded by saying:

> Frankly, hospital administrators don't make policy like this but that's one I would love to make. If I could, I would absolutely forbid every obstetrician from doing an episiotomy. Forbid it. Absolutely. For a very simple reason, because I know that by doing that not only would I insure the revenue strength of this hospital immediately because of what's going to happen when a gal tears herself from stem to stern and we have to respond with major surgical procedures and lots of blood and prolonged stay in the hospital. But I know also that ten years down the road that woman is going to come back in to have everything put back in place.

What is striking about this comment is not only the absolute derision which this administrator expresses toward the women who pay to give birth at this hospital, but also the certainty with which he predicts extremely unlikely outcomes. There is a lack of evidence that routine episiotomy prevents either perineal trauma or pelvic floor relaxation, but there is evidence which associates perineal trauma with episiotomy (Edwards and Waldorf, 1984, p. 143).

Martin (1987) discusses some forms of resistance which women use to avoid unwanted treatment by doctors and hospital staff. Women sometimes conceal what is happening to them. When they go into labor, they do not share this information with anyone until they are unable to conceal their labor any longer. By doing this they can avoid arriving at the hospital too soon, thereby increasing their chances of avoiding unnecessary interventions, including Cesarean section. Some women go for long walks around the hospital and do not return for hours. Other women resist by unstrapping electronic fetal monitors. One woman told of how she used physical force to avoid an episiotomy:

> I catch a glimpse of the flash of metal (the delivery room scissors for an episiotomy) going past me. We had done perineal massage every night

(to make the perineum flexible enough to avoid tearing or the need for an episiotomy). I grabbed the scissors; from the home birth I knew it took seventeen minutes to sterilize them. I wasn't even trying to take them out of the doctor's hand. It wasn't a logical thought at the time. I was just trying to break the sterile field. I said, "You aren't cutting me," and asked him to massage, but he didn't know how. He just went like this [gestures halfheartedly] and [after the baby emerged] said, "Well, you tore!" He wanted me to tear. (Martin, 1987, pp. 142–143)

Home birth is, of course, the ultimate form of resistance. By staying at home, birthing women refuse to participate in a system in which power and control rest in the hands of physicians and in which birthing women are marginalized.

Dwinnell (1992) argues that the treatment which many women receive at the hands of doctors in hospitals is a form of violence against women. Some of the manifestations of violence by doctors include (1) doing vaginal exams and other procedures without explaining to the woman what is being done or asking her permission; (2) telling a woman she is hurting her fetus if she questions or refuses tests or procedures which the doctor sees as necessary; (3) threatening to use various tests, procedures, or drugs if the woman does not cooperate, maintain control, or birth fast enough; and (4) using intimidation supported by professional status.

Despite the treatment which many women receive from doctors in the hospital, and the resistance which some women demonstrate, the fact remains that most women continue to birth in hospitals with doctors in attendance. As mentioned earlier, according to Jordan, 80 percent of birthing women receive epidural anesthesia and 80 percent of all labors are augmented with Pitocin. (These two statistics are not unrelated, since epidurals often have the effect of slowing down labor. These labors are then speeded up with Pitocin.) Episiotomies are done in over 90 percent of all first-time births. The most common position for birth continues to be the lithotomy position in which the woman is flat on her back with her legs spread apart and her feet in stirrups. Most pregnant women experience at least two ultrasound scans during a pregnancy. Most women over thirty-five have testing done to check for genetic abnormalities in the fetus (Jordan, 1993, p. 143). The question, then, is how is the participation of women within the medical model maintained?

Jordan (1993, pp. 142–143) sheds some interesting light on this question. Jordan first wrote *Birth in Four Cultures* in 1978. In the first edition of the book she talked about birth in U.S. culture and the extent to which it was defined and shaped by high technology and the power and authority of the medical profession. Jordan predicted then that over time birth would become less technologized and more responsive to the needs of women, resulting in increased maternal satisfaction. In a revised edition of the book published in 1993, Jordan talks about being surprised by the fact that over the fifteen-year period between 1978 and 1993, medicalization and technologization of American births have intensified. To be sure, there have been changes over the years. Many family-centered perinatal care programs have been introduced: many hospitals now have birthing rooms, and even more have combined labor-delivery-recovery rooms, so that women do not have to be moved from one environment to the next during and after the birth. Most hospitals offer childbirth education classes, and many require women and their partners to take them.

The increased technologization of birth in the United States has been mediated, Jordan argues, by a willingness on the part of the medical profession to treat laboring women (in particular, those who have been properly socialized through hospital-based childbirth education classes) as people to interact with, rather than as bodies to be acted upon. Technologization has increased along with childbirth education which completely prepares women for a technologized birth. Through childbirth education classes many women have been socialized to accept and expect the technocratic model of birth and the authority of the physician which this model implies.

CHILDBIRTH AS A FEATURE OF SOCIAL RELATIONS

Rothman (1989) argues that what we know about birth has been determined by the way it is managed. While in our society we believe that medicine has a monopoly over the management of childbirth because childbirth is a medical event, it may be, rather, that childbirth is a medical event because of the medical monopoly over the management of childbirth. As mentioned before, research demonstrates that the use of routine childbirth procedures cannot be justified based upon scientific evidence regarding their effectiveness.

In order, then, to understand the medical model of childbirth it is important to understand that technologies and the circumstances which determine their use do not arise by themselves but are features of social relations (Jordan, 1993, 1980; Rothman, 1989, 1982; Martin, 1987). Braverman (1974) and Margolin (1974) have made this argument in relation to technology in the workplace, but it can be extended to other areas as well. In relation to childbirth, for example, Rich (1986) argues that forceps effectively displaced midwives through a male monopoly over that invention. Rich (1986), Arms (1975), and others discuss the development of childbirth practices (the use of forceps, the lithotomy position, and more recent technologies including drugs and monitoring devices) as products of the relationship between physician and patient.

Such technologies serve the interests of the physicians by making births more convenient and expedient to attend and by reinforcing their position of authority. Ehrenreich and English (1979), Rothman (1982, 1989), Martin (1987), Davis-Floyd (1992), and Jordan (1993) take this argument one step further and relate the current situation regarding childbirth and the role of women in medicine to the larger political economy in which these phenomena are located. The definition of childbirth as a risk-filled, potentially life-threatening event leads many women to fear childbirth. They seek out the medical model because it promises the most scientifically and technologically advanced methods and procedures for insuring a safe birth. Scientific evidence does not support the routine use of many of the standard hospital practices and procedures, yet these persist. In Jordan's words, "What we need to keep in mind here is that birthing systems themselves are part of a larger cultural system, the articulation of which takes place within an economic and political structure via the socialization of birth participants, and via birth conceptualizations' location within the society's larger ideological system" (Jordan, 1980, p. 73).

The complexity (or at least the belief in the complexity) of technological questions, apparatus, and so on, has led to a reliance on the authority of experts on technological issues, resulting in a dichotomy between layperson and expert. As technology encroaches further and further into areas that are personal in nature, individuals relinquish more and more of their autonomy to experts, even in the most intimate areas of their lives. People are rendered incompetent to make decisions about their personal conditions and unable to fully experience the pleasure and pain of being human (Illich, 1976).

With respect to childbirth specifically, Harrison argues that the issue is one of authority and control, not one of method. While there are numerous problems and risks associated with dominant childbirth practices, the authority of medical experts in relation to birthing women remains problematic regardless of any change in dominant practices. Harrison recalls that when she was a resident in obstetrics and gynecology a new paper came out on the benefits of walking during labor and she left a copy around for her colleagues in labor and delivery to read. As she thought about the paper she suddenly had visions of obstetricians deciding that all women should ambulate during labor, and of laboring women being forced to march up and down hospital halls. The problem is that doctors decide how women should labor and give birth. Women have little or no control over their experience (Harrison, 1982, p. 178).

The medical model reflects the values of a capitalist society in which everything is commodified. Babies are defined as products. Women are viewed as laborers, the producers of products. The role of technology is to insure the quality of the product. But the laborer controls neither the process of production nor the outcome (Rothman, 1989; Martin, 1987).

The specific circumstances of hospital births will vary. Some physicians are more willing to work with their "patients" than others. Some institutions have more flexible rules and policies than others. What remains true in every instance, however, is that within the hospital setting, control rests in the hands of the medical personnel who work within the parameters set by the administrative rules of the institution. Physicians exercise a virtual monopoly over attending women in childbirth and of defining standards of treatment.

Tew (1990) argues that every culture has its own medicine men on whom it relies to solve its problems of illness and death. In contemporary Western culture it is academically trained doctors who enjoy this status.

Physicians in relation to patients have what Starr (1992) has termed "cultural authority": the authority to interpret symptoms, diagnose illness, and prescribe treatment. Cultural authority is tied to technocratic ideology that marginalizes the experience of birthing women. Physicians shape the patient's understanding of her own experience and by doing so "create the conditions under which their advice seems appropriate" (Starr, 1982, p. 14). Physicians usually do not have the power to force patients to accept their interpretation of symptoms or to follow their advice. As discussed earlier, with respect to childbirth there are instances where physicians have sought the assistance of the courts to coerce women to accept both the medical interpretation of the situation as well as the medically recommended course of action. In these cases, the state has intervened on behalf of the fetus, to order that women undergo Cesarean sections against their will (Rothman, 1989, p. 195). Under more typical circumstances, however, women follow the advice and directions of physicians not because of the threat of coercion, but out of fear of the consequences of ignoring medical authority (Starr, 1982).

The medical model claims to offer the only responsible way to give birth. Deviations from this model are viewed as being fraught with risk. Physicians present themselves and are established as the only practitioners who can provide competent care for birthing women. From the perspective of the medical model, midwives are viewed as lesser practitioners who are unable to provide the level of skill and expertise available from physicians.

4

The Midwifery Approach
to Birth

> You are a midwife: you are assisting at someone else's birth. Do good without show or fuss. Facilitate what is happening rather than what you think ought to be happening. If you must take the lead, lead so that the mother is helped yet still free and in charge. When the baby is born the mother will rightly say, "We did it ourselves!"
>
> —*Tao Te Ching*, written 2500 years ago,
> quoted in Sheila Kitzinger, *The Midwife Challenge*, p. 1

The medical model is part of our cultural consciousness. It is difficult for most people to imagine birth unencumbered by machines and painkilling medication. It is even harder to imagine birth taking place without a physician in attendance, especially outside of a hospital setting.

The medical model, however, is not the only model for birth. The midwifery model offers a different philosophy of birth and consequently different practices as well. From the perspective of the midwifery model, childbirth is viewed as a healthy activity and as an important event in the lives of women and their families. During pregnancy and birth, women require physical care involving examination and screening, but they also require social and emotional support and comfort for this personal event. Throughout pregnancy and birth, midwives act as teachers and guides for pregnant women. In the midwifery model, birth is something that women do, not something that is done to them. The midwifery model offers a view of childbirth which is woman-centered. Women give birth, and midwives assist them in doing so.

This chapter examines the midwifery approach to birth and looks at the relationship between this approach and the medical model. In addition, the chapter discusses various types of midwives and the professional relationships which exist among them. The relationship between the midwifery approach and the medical model raises important questions about law and professional autonomy which midwives face. There are also important questions about institutional control which are explored through the case of nurse-midwifery associates. The final section of the chapter discusses the concept of the free-standing birth center and describes how issues surrounding such birth centers reflect the legal, professional, and institutional control questions addressed in the chapter as a whole.

THE MIDWIFERY MODEL

In the midwifery model, the experiential knowledge of birthing women is seen as equally important as, or more important than, technical knowledge. What women know through their bodies is neither discounted nor ignored. Talking, touching, laughing, crying, and other forms of communication are encouraged and, indeed, are central to the birthing activity. The physical and emotional health of the mother is seen as essential for the health of the baby. Babies and mothers are viewed as one unit, and mothers are not considered threats to their babies.

In the midwifery model, midwives and mothers work closely together. Midwives become an intimate part of the birthing process. Oakley and Houd offer a clear example in this description of labor: "The woman gets on her knees. The midwife is sitting in front of her, also on her knees. The woman puts her head on the midwife's shoulder, who then holds her head in her hands. They are finding a rhythm together" (Oakley and Houd, 1990, p. 72).

Page (1988) identifies five principles which should characterize modern midwifery care. The first of these, continuity of care, is essential to midwifery because it allows midwives to get to know the women they serve. A relationship of trust develops and the birth becomes a shared celebration. Continuity also aids in the ability to make accurate clinical judgments because midwives get to know the mother's history, her current state of health, and the physical and emotional strength of the family. Continuity of care provides the foundation for accountability, which, Page argues, is an important factor in developing professional autonomy for midwifery.

The second principle which Page identifies is respect for the normal. Because midwives approach birth with a confidence in and respect for the physiological process of birth, they avoid routine intervention. This reluctance to intervene in the physiological process of birth represents a rejection of technocratic ideology. It runs directly contrary to the technocratic approach, which assumes that nature must be dominated and controlled. The practice of midwifery is based upon prevention, which from this perspective is broadly defined to include the many aspects of life which affect well-being, including the provision of food, shelter, and income. As a result, midwives are often involved in the formation of social policy and in outreach programs for communities of women who are particularly in need.

In the case of complicated pregnancies, however, when intervention may be necessary, midwives provide a source of emotional support and can work along with obstetricians to provide care. By constantly teaching and explaining, midwives fulfill the third principle which Page discusses: enabling women to make informed choices about medical care. Even when the situation warrants technological intervention, the midwife can act as an advocate for birthing women and families, maintaining an emphasis on the human aspects of birth. Midwives serve as advisors and guides for birthing women.

Fourth, midwives recognize birth as more than a medical event. Many authors talk about the importance which midwives attach to the emotional and social aspects of birth in addition to the physical aspects. Birth is physical, but it is also emotional, spiritual, and sexual. The tradition of midwifery has demonstrated a sensitivity to all the aspects of birth. Midwives work to see that parents are able to experience the fullness of birth.

Finally, midwifery offers family-centered care which recognizes the diversity of families. Families come in a variety of forms and from a variety of backgrounds. Their members have different personalities, different upbringings, and differing expectations about the birth. The continuity of care which is part of the midwifery model can help midwives to meet the needs of both birthing women and their families.

The midwifery model offers an alternative to the "risk approach" toward pregnancy and birth by focusing instead on what Oakley and Houd call primary prevention. "The meaning of the concept of primary prevention in relation to pregnancy and birth is that it is essentially a question of strengthening the woman to give birth and take care of her own baby. The mother is the central person in maternity care, and the midwife, the doctor, and other health workers are her assistants" (Oakley and Houd, 1990, p. 128). Primary prevention, then, is based not upon surveillance and control, but rather upon the desire to offer support and to meet the needs of each individual birthing woman within a variety of circumstances.

Rothman believes that midwifery—working with the women in labor to create a birth experience that meets their needs—is feminist praxis. The medical monopoly regarding childbirth has meant defining childbirth in medical terms, leaving out other factors. By doing so we limit our understanding of birth.

What midwifery offers us is not just tossing in a few social or psychological variables, but a reconceptualization of the "facts" of procreation.
A profession controls not only people—as doctors control the nurses
who "follow orders"; the patients who "comply"—more important, a
profession controls the development of knowledge. In regard to birth,
the profession of medicine determines who may attend a birth or what
birth attendants may do, but it controls also what we know of birth
itself. (Rothman, 1989, pp. 172–173)

What midwifery offers, then, is not simply a gentler birth in prettier sur-
roundings, but rather an alternative conception which offers nothing less than
a different understanding of birth itself. With this new understanding, many
of what were formerly understood as "facts" of birth come to be seen as
"artifacts" of the medical model (Rothman, 1989; Jordan, 1993; Oakley and
Houd, 1990).

Rothman (1989, pp. 179–181) identifies a number of these artifacts. It is
commonly believed, for example, that nausea and vomiting are a common
part of labor. Midwives who have not limited the food or drink intake of
laboring women report much less nausea and vomiting. It is not clear, then,
whether nausea and vomiting are a result of labor or of lack of food. But the
medical model attributes these symptoms to labor, rendering them conditions
to be treated. The "fact" that nausea and vomiting are a routine symptom of
labor becomes an artifact because its meaning is constructed through the
medical approach.

The medical model also maintains that infection is likely to occur if much
time passes after the amniotic sac has been broken and before birth occurs.
The questions are, How likely is infection? What are the most likely sources
of infection? Are there ways to prevent infections? Jane Dwinnell, a nurse-
midwife, tells some of the stories of the many births she has attended in her
book *Birth Stories* (1992). One of them is about Kitty, who gave birth in a
hospital-based birthing center. Kitty was expecting her first child when her
membranes ruptured at thirty-seven weeks. It was not until four days later
that Kitty gave birth. Three of those days were spent at the birthing center.
During that time, the staff would check her temperature and the baby's heart
rate, but internal exams were avoided until Kitty was in active labor and nearly
fully dilated. Dwinnell argues that there is no need for birth to occur within
twenty-four hours after the membranes have ruptured as long as there are not
signs of infection. The absence of internal exams reduces the likelihood of
infection.

A third common belief is that breast milk does not come in for three days
after birth. When mothers have access to their babies and can breastfeed

regularly, milk comes in within twenty-four to forty-eight hours. Palmer (1988) discusses a number of medically supported beliefs and practices which undermine the ability of women to breastfeed. Advising women to schedule feedings, limiting the time the baby spends at the breast, and using supplementary feedings of sugar water or formula all interfere with milk production. Even physicians who are generally supportive of breastfeeding can behave in ways which undermine the ability of women to breastfeed successfully. Both of my children were large and healthy at birth. My son weighed 9 pounds, 11 ounces, and was nearly 23 inches long. My daughter weighed 8 pounds, 11 ounces, and was 21 and ½ inches long. They were both exclusively breastfed for their first six months, and they both gained weight slowly and steadily and showed no signs of being nutritionally deprived in any way. With my son, his doctor wanted him brought into the office once a week for weighing because he was a breastfed baby. In my daughter's case, her doctor felt that she was not gaining weight rapidly enough and warned me about inadequate milk supply.

Despite this lack of support, I was able to breastfeed my children for quite some time: my son until he was two, and my daughter until she was three. But my experiences with the medical profession over this issue are not unique. Women say all the time that they stopped nursing because they did not have enough milk. Palmer (1988) says that to this day "insufficient milk" is the most common reason that women give for abandoning breastfeeding. Breastfeeding poses a significant challenge to the technocratic world view and the desire for order and control which it implies. When women breastfeed, the amount of milk the baby ingests can be neither seen nor measured. The production of breast milk cannot be controlled by artificial means. Breastfeeding is relational and reciprocal. It is something mothers and babies do together. It is the baby's suckling which in large part determines the amount of milk produced.

A fourth artifact is the belief that when birthing women are fully dilated, the pushing stage of labor begins. If it does not, this is a sign of pathology known as "second stage arrest." Midwives practicing outside the medical model sometimes find that women reach full dilation and then roll over and fall asleep. After a rest, the labor starts up again and birth occurs, without intervention. It is unlikely that this would happen within the medical model, however, because the rest period probably would be seen as pathological and would be treated.

PROFESSIONAL AUTONOMY AND THE ROLE OF LAW

Moving away from the medical model would allow us to see birth in other ways. The midwifery model offers the possibility of new understanding based upon a different philosophy and different practices. If we demedicalize childbirth, then the medical profession loses its monopoly over the management of childbirth in the United States (Rothman, 1989). But the politics which surround the medical model do, of course, complicate the issue. The authority of doctors within the medical professions has given them the power to control and sometimes block alternatives to the medical model of birth and, in other cases, to influence the shape alternatives will take and the circumstances under which they will exist.

In order to understand how this is accomplished, it is necessary to consider the characteristics of a profession. A profession is an occupation which has acquired or has convinced others that it has acquired certain characteristics including (1) a body of theoretical knowledge obtained through extensive study; (2) altruism or service orientation; (3) autonomy in controlling the profession, including selecting and training new members, establishing a code of ethics, and disciplining its own members; (4) authority over clients who are thought to be unable to judge their own needs; (5) a distinctive occupational culture; and (6) recognition in the law and by the community that the occupation is a profession (Stromberg, 1988, p. 206). It is important to note, as Stromberg points out, that professions may vary with regard to these characteristics. What is significant for a profession is having the power to convince others that it has these characteristics and therefore deserves a monopoly over practice (Stromberg, 1988, p. 207).

Among the medical professions, physicians enjoy the highest professional status. No group of midwives enjoys comparable status and the autonomy it brings. It is important to say that not all midwives see themselves as practicing medicine or as vying for a place in the medical hierarchy. In this society, however, attending women in childbirth is viewed as practicing medicine, so all midwives are placed within this hierarchy, regardless of how they view themselves. The organization of medical professions leads to different statuses and responsibilities among midwives.

Different groups of midwives do, indeed, view themselves differently. In their practice a distinction is made among (1) certified nurse-midwives; (2) lay, empirical, or independent midwives; and (3) direct-entry midwives. Certified nurse-midwives (CNMs) are nurses who have received advanced training in midwifery and are certified by the American College of Nurse-Midwives. In all but a few states certification of nurse-midwives is recognized in the laws governing the practice of nurse-midwifery (Bidgood-Wilson, Barickman, and Ackley, 1992). They practice in hospitals, free-standing birth centers, and sometimes at home.

Lay, empirical, or independent midwives learn midwifery through an apprenticeship to an experienced midwife. Direct-entry midwives, like lay midwives, do not come to midwifery through a background in nursing, but they have completed a course of training that meets the requirements for state licensing (Kitzinger, 1988, p. 40; Myers-Ciecko, 1988, p. 63). Many states, however, do not have provisions for licensing direct-entry midwives. Lay midwives and direct-entry midwives usually attend births at home. It is important to note that sometimes the terms lay, empirical, independent, and direct-entry midwives are used interchangeably.

No group of midwives enjoys the legal status of physicians, who are consistently recognized in every state as having the legal right to attend women in childbirth. Yet the law does distinguish between nurse-midwives and other midwives. Virtually every state allows nurse-midwives to attend women in childbirth. But about half of the states require nurse-midwives to have an alliance with a physician, for the purposes of backup services and oversight. Lay and direct-entry midwives find themselves in very different legal circumstances from one state to the next. In some states, their practice is legal, in others it is illegal, and in still others it is not mentioned in the law. (Sullivan and Weitz, 1988; Bidgood-Wilson, Barickman, and Ackley, 1992).

All midwives are commonly viewed as less well trained and less competent than physicians, but this view can be attributed in part to the power of the medical model, which distorts what is known and what can be seen about midwifery practice. In fact, researchers have found evidence that contradicts the common view. A study of nearly twelve thousand births in free-standing birth centers, where most births are attended by nurse-midwives, showed very little intervention and excellent outcomes (Rooks et al., 1989). A study done by Lewis Mehl in 1977 compared 1,046 planned home births with 1,046 planned hospital births and found home births, which are usually attended by midwives, to be safer than hospital births (Mehl, 1978). More recent studies on home birth show similar positive outcomes (Sullivan and Weitz, 1988).

Gender is also an important factor in determining the status of both groups of midwives. As Sullivan and Weitz argue, "The male gender of most physicians significantly increases their credibility and lobbying power in the legal and judicial systems which continue to be dominated by men. At the same time, the female gender of most midwives works against them. Moreover, the fact that it is women who are encroaching on their occupational turf appears to threaten physicians' egos and heighten their hostility" (Sullivan and Weitz, 1988, p. 94). The issue of gender is even more heightened in the case of nurse-midwives, since nursing developed as an ancillary occupation providing support for physicians, under the direction of physicians and hospital administrators. Nursing developed as a female-dominated occupation with a female image. As a result, nurses are made even more vulnerable than women in general to sex stereotyping and sex discrimination (Stromberg, 1988, pp. 208–209).

The status of nurse-midwives creates a dilemma. Because of their legal status as medical professionals and their direct links to physicians as well as to some health care institutions, nurse-midwives enjoy greater legitimacy in the culture and in the law than do lay or direct-entry midwives. As a result, nurse-midwives sometimes seek to distance themselves from other midwives. During a debate over midwifery legislation in Vermont, a nurse-midwife said, "One of the problems now is that you can't differentiate who the lay people are, who the professional people are, and what the nurse-midwife is" (Teasley, 1986, p. 269). In the state where I did my own research, there is virtually no interaction between nurse-midwives and other midwives. Lay midwifery and direct-entry midwifery are illegal in the state, and nurse-midwives have no interest in jeopardizing their own somewhat vulnerable standing by networking with midwives who operate outside the law.

Relations between nurse-midwives and lay and direct-entry midwives are sometimes more cooperative. The Midwives Alliance of North America (MANA) was formed in April 1982. The purposes of the organization include (1) expanding communication and support among North American midwives (including Canadian midwives), (2) promoting guidelines for the education and training of midwives, (3) promoting midwifery as a quality health care option for women and their families, (4) promoting research in the field of midwifery care, and (5) establishing a link between midwives and other professional and nonprofessional groups concerned with the health of women and their families (Ashford, 1983, p. 101). Membership in MANA is open to all midwives, students, and supporters of midwifery.

While there are nurse-midwives who are members of MANA, there has been very little official communication between MANA and the American College of Nurse-Midwives (ACNM) (Myers-Ciecko, 1988). In recent years, though, the ACNM has shown an interest in coalition building, which is reflected in an ongoing discussion of three questions:

1. Should the American College of Nurse-Midwives accredit educational programs for midwives which do not require nursing as a prerequisite?

2. Should graduates of such programs sit for the American College of Nurse-Midwives exam?

3. If the group should say yes to these first two questions, should the American College of Nurse-Midwives then extend membership to non-nurse-midwives?

The ACNM continues to discuss these controversial questions, although they have not yet been resolved. An affirmative answer would change the nature of the ACNM as a body and would also raise some interesting legal issues in the many states where the law makes a clear distinction between nurse-midwives and non-nurse-midwives. Consideration of these questions, however, indicates an awareness of the need for midwives to network across barriers and differences in order to strengthen their profession.

At the same time that nurse-midwives derive some benefit from their status as health professionals and their links to physicians, these same things lock them into an inferior status in relation to physicians. As Rothman argues, "It may be that nurse-midwife is a contradiction in terms, with an inherent dilemma. Nurses, in our medical system, are defined by their relationship to doctors, and midwives are, in the meaning of the term derived from Old English, 'with the woman.' Nurse-midwives operating in the medical establishment have a hard time as 'advocates of the childbearing couple.' The essential elements of cooption—job, prestige, professional recognition—are all right there" (Rothman, 1982, p. 73).

The situation of the midwives I have studied is a case in point. As mentioned before, lay and direct-entry midwives practice outside the law in the state where I studied. Nurse-midwives stand on much firmer legal footing. They are recognized as health professionals who can practice as long as they have an alliance with a physician(s) who can provide obstetrical support. The major medical center in the state offers no practicing privileges to nurse-midwives, but some small hospitals in the state have offered privileges to a few nurse-midwives. The professional autonomy of nurse-midwives is limited. Doctors and hospital administrators exercise a great deal of control over their ability to practice and over the circumstances under which they may practice. Often, efforts on the part of nurses or nurse-midwives to increase their professional autonomy are met with opposition from physicians' organizations which try to block or coopt such efforts. In July 1994, the governor signed legislation allowing the board of nursing to credential and license nurses as "advanced practice nurses." The board of nursing was also given the authority to establish rules and regulations which would guide advanced practice nursing. This legislation includes nurse-midwives but is not specific to them. During debate over the legislation, the medical society in the state contacted all of its members by mail, outlining the intent of the legislation and encouraging members to actively oppose it. They did manage to have one scheduled vote tabled, and the legislation which ultimately passed is a revised version which reflects at least some of the concerns of the doctors that nurses not be given so much autonomy. In most states nurse-practitioners and advanced practice nurses do have the legal right to govern their own practice and to engage in practices which they were formerly prohibited from doing, such as prescribing drugs and admitting patients to hospitals. Yet

within the medical hierarchy, physicians still enjoy greater status and autonomy, which allows them to continue to influence the degree of professional
autonomy afforded to nurses and nurse-midwives.

Current Medicaid policy offers an example of the effects of physicians'
power and status. Medicaid has set reimbursement of CNM services at 65
percent of the physician reimbursement rate. Some insurance companies have
started to use the same formula for determining reimbursement. This takes
away the right of nurse-midwives to set their own fees. In many instances,
this will jeopardize the practices of nurse-midwives and will threaten facilities
such as free-standing birth centers which are usually run by nurse-midwives.

In 1994 legislation was introduced in the U.S. Senate and House of
Representatives which would have overridden this policy. The Primary Care
Health Practitioner Act set the Medicaid reimbursement rate for certified
nurse-midwives, nurse-practitioners, and clinical nurse specialists (CNSs) at
97 percent of the physician payment rate. The legislation clearly represents
an improvement over current policy, but it still makes the payment rate for
nurse-midwives a function of the rates set by physicians. This legislation was
reintroduced in 1995 with some significant changes: There is no specific
mention of nurse-midwives in the legislation and the reimbursement rate for
nurse-practitioners and CNSs is set at 85 percent of the physician rate.

The issue of the professional autonomy of midwives needs to be addressed. It may be that professional autonomy for midwives requires
severing links to the medical system. This, of course, is not easy to do
because of the need for networking and backup services as well as because
of the legal issues. The authority of the physician is not rooted merely in
cultural conditioning and expectation; it is also defined by law. Physicians
are the only medical practitioners who are consistently recognized in every
state as having legal authority to attend women in childbirth. In contrast,
the marginality of midwifery is suggested by the absence of any unified
body of law that regulates it.

Regardless of the specific provisions of the law in any particular state, lay
midwives, direct-entry midwives, and nurse-midwives often face strong
opposition from the medical establishment. Their uncertain legal status
contributes markedly to their vulnerability. The following examples show
that this opposition is widespread and takes a variety of forms.

Since the mid-1970s, several lay midwives in California have been arrested,
while others have been faced with active investigations. Most of the arrests
were based upon claims of incompetence brought by physicians against the
midwives (Ashford, 1986, p. 8). Included among these cases is that of Rosalie
Tarpening, a licensed physical therapist and lay midwife. Tarpening said that
she was the primary attendant at 354 deliveries over a nine-year period, with

no perinatal deaths and no hospital transfers for mothers or newborns. In 1979, Tarpening was arrested following the death of Gabriel Villa, whose birth she had attended (Sullivan and Weitz, 1988, p. 84). Though the delivery was an easy one, the baby was clearly in trouble at birth. Tarpening tried resuscitation but with no positive result. She immediately sent the baby to Madera Community Hospital, where the infant was pronounced dead in the emergency room.

Tarpening was initially charged with first-degree murder (which carries a mandatory death sentence in California), practicing medicine without a license, and grand theft for charging for her services. The prosecution argued that Tarpening was responsible for the death because she had mismanaged the labor which resulted in insufficient oxygen for the baby. The defense argued that the baby's death had been caused by physicians at Madera Community Hospital when they pumped too much air at too great a pressure into the baby's lungs in their resuscitation attempt. The trial testimony by pathologist Edith Potter supported the defense argument. Eventually, the murder charges were dropped due to lack of evidence of malicious intent. Tarpening was then tried and convicted of one misdemeanor count of practicing medicine without a license. No expert witnesses were allowed to testify about the safety of home birth. Tarpening received a one-year suspended sentence. She also had her physical therapist license suspended for six months (Edwards and Waldorf, 1984, pp. 171–172; Sullivan and Weitz, 1988, pp. 84–85).

In Arizona, where lay midwifery is legal, lay midwives have reported harassment by physicians. The law requires that home birth clients see a physician once a month during pregnancy, and midwives often accompany their clients on these visits. The midwives report that physicians often punish clients for having home births. This punishment might take the form of verbal reprimands, but in other cases midwives have claimed that doctors inflict unnecessary pain on home birth clients during examination and treatment. One midwife, for example, took a client to the hospital following a home birth in order for the client to have a minor vaginal tear repaired. The emergency room doctor refused to give the client anesthesia for her stitches because she had had a home birth (Weitz and Sullivan, 1986).

In Vermont there are no laws regarding lay midwifery except a requirement that birth certificates be filed. Attending childbirth is not considered the practice of medicine unless drugs are administered. In 1981, charges were brought against a lay midwife who administered Pitocin and then ergotrate to stop a hemorrhage. Although this case did go to trial, the "Good Samaritan" Law was used to gain acquittal since the birth in this case was unattended and the midwife was called only when problems developed (Sallomi, Pallow-Fleury, and McMahon, 1982, p. 25).

INSTITUTIONAL CONTROL: THE CASE OF
NURSE-MIDWIFERY ASSOCIATES

While nurse-midwives are on somewhat firmer legal footing than other midwives, they are faced with a great deal of opposition from physicians. This opposition is manifested in a variety of ways, including refusal to grant hospital privileges to nurse-midwives, refusal to provide the backup support which is commonly required in order for nurse-midwives to practice, and efforts to increase the amount of physician oversight of midwifery practice.

The case of Nurse-Midwifery Associates serves as a prime example of the power of institutional control (*Nurse-Midwifery Associates vs. Henderson Community Hospital and Southern Hills Hospital*, Petition for Writ of Certiorari, U.S. District Court of Appeals, Sixth Circuit, October 1990). Susan Sizemore and Victoria Henderson had been practicing nurse-midwives in Tennessee for a number of years. In January, 1980 the two formed Nurse-Midwifery Associates (NMA), a private-sector nurse-midwifery service. Sizemore and Henderson entered into an arrangement with Dr. Darrell Martin, who agreed to provide medical supervision and services. NMA clients would give birth in a hospital setting. Sizemore and Henderson applied for practicing privileges at Hendersonville Community Hospital (HCH), a small, privately owned community hospital in Hendersonville, Tennessee, where Martin was a member of the medical staff.

HCH was initially very receptive to Henderson and Sizemore. The nurse-midwives developed a protocol along with Dr. Martin. The applications for practicing privileges were approved by the HCH department of obstetrics and gynecology pending approval of the protocol. After being approved by the ob-gyn department, the protocol was sent on to the departments of anesthesia and pediatrics. Anesthesia approved the protocol. The department of pediatrics, however, unanimously voted to deny privileges to Henderson and Sizemore because of concerns about their proposed practice. Discussion continued over the issue, and meetings were held to address the pediatricians' concerns. The pediatricians continued to refuse to approve the protocol. Some pediatricians threatened to leave if they were required to see newborns whose births had been attended by Sizemore and Henderson.

In the meantime, Sizemore and Henderson had obtained a bank loan of fifty thousand dollars based upon the hospital's initial positive response. They began setting up their practice. In the end, however, the pediatrics department refused to change its position, and Sizemore and Henderson were denied practicing privileges at HCH.

Prior to any final decision by HCH, the nurse-midwives applied for privileges at Southern Hills Hospital (SHH), also a privately owned community hospital. Initial discussions with the hospital administrator were positive. The executive committee of the hospital appointed an ad hoc committee to review the applications. No minutes were kept of the meetings held by the ad hoc committee. While the ad hoc committee was formulating its decision, it became clear that a number of doctors at SHH were strongly opposed to granting privileges to Sizemore and Henderson. Dr. Stephen Melkin, a member of the hospital's executive committee, told Martin, "If nurse-midwives started delivering babies, the next thing they would want to do is heart surgery" (*Nurse-Midwifery Associates*, p. 9). The ad hoc committee recommended that Sizemore and Henderson be denied privileges, and the executive committee approved their recommendation. On October 16, 1980, the board of trustees denied the applications for privileges but said that Sizemore and Henderson could reapply if certain conditions were met. These conditions included requirements that two obstetricians with practicing privileges at SHH supervise Sizemore and Henderson and that an obstetrician be present for all births.

After Sizemore and Henderson were informed of the board of trustees' decision, they indicated that they would reapply for privileges and would address the recommendations of the ad hoc committee. At that point, Sizemore and Henderson were told by Dr. George Andrews, chair of obstetrics and gynecology at SHH, that if they were to reapply, the obstetrics department would adopt new policies regarding mandatory enemas, perineal shaving, electronic fetal monitoring, intravenous fluids, and ambulation, and would close the birthing room. In November 1980, the decision was made to close the birthing room at SHH. This precluded Sizemore, Henderson, and Martin from initiating their practice.

Sizemore and Henderson had also applied for privileges at Vanderbilt University Hospital. Prior to any decision from Vanderbilt, conversations took place among Dr. Lonnie S. Burnett, chairman of the department of obstetrics and gynecology at Vanderbilt; Dr. Frank Boehm, a member of the Vanderbilt ob-gyn department; and Dr. B. K. Hibbett, an obstetrician with privileges at Vanderbilt who had previously been head of ob-gyn at Baptist Hospital in Nashville and who remained an important member of the ob-gyn staff. Dr. Hibbett was a strong opponent of nurse-midwifery. All of the doctors deny that they discussed the issue of nurse-midwifery or the applications of Sizemore and Henderson. It was certainly important, however, that good relations be maintained between Vanderbilt and Baptist Hospitals. They had the largest maternity services in the area, there was considerable overlap among their ob-gyn staffs, and Vanderbilt's ob-gyn residents were permitted to rotate through Baptist Hospital as part of their training. On September 2, 1980, Vanderbilt denied privileges to the nurse-midwives.

In addition, problems began to develop regarding malpractice coverage for Dr. Darrell Martin, who was insured by State Volunteer Mutual Insurance Company (SVMIC). In the early 1980s, SVMIC insured nearly 80 percent of all physicians in Tennessee and was organized under the auspices of the Tennessee Medical Association (TMA). According to Sizemore, Henderson, and Martin, TMA was opposed to the expanded use of nurse-midwives.

Martin informed SVMIC in June 1980 that he would be leaving his practice and would be working with NMA. SVMIC's underwriter contacted Martin and asked for clarification about his relationship with NMA and for any other information pertinent to their risk as his insurance provider. Hibbett was a member of the SVMIC board of directors as well as of the claims review committee. An obstetrical nurse at Baptist Hospital reported having a conversation with Hibbett in which he told her that they (SVMIC) were going to get Martin's insurance and set nurse-midwifery back twenty years. An obstetrician at Baptist Hospital recalled a similar conversation with Hibbett.

The underwriting committee of SVMIC concluded that Martin's relationship to NMA increased the financial risks to the insurance company and recommended that his coverage be canceled. In October 1980, the board of directors of SVMIC concurred with the recommendation and voted unanimously not to renew Martin's malpractice coverage. This left Sizemore and Henderson with no physician backup. They were unable to locate another physician willing to work with them and were forced to close their nurse-midwifery practice.

On March 2, 1981, Sizemore, Henderson, Martin, and two clients, Richard and Margaret Carpenter, filed a complaint in the United States District Court for the middle district of Tennessee, seeking damages under the provisions of the Sherman Antitrust Act. Those named in the suit included HCH and Dr. Conrad Shackleford; SHH and Drs. Stephen Melkin, Harry Baer, and George Andrews; Vanderbilt University Hospital; SVMIC; and Dr. B. K. Hibbett. The suit alleged that these persons and institutions conspired to restrain competition. The alleged conspiracies were (1) among HCH, Shackleford, and other members of the HCH pediatrics staff; (2) among SHH and Melkin, Baer, and Andrews; (3) between Vanderbilt and the members of its medical staff; (4) between Vanderbilt and Hibbett; (5) between HCH and SHH; and (6) between SVMIC and Hibbett.

The questions which the case raised were these:

1. "Whether as a matter of law, a trial court is precluded from finding that a hospital conspired with members of its medical staff to restrain trade in violation of Section I of the Sherman Act by denying staff

privileges to practitioners in potential competition with those staff members."

2. "Whether a hospital can be vicariously liable under Section I of the Sherman Act for a decision by its medical staff denying staff privileges to practitioners in potential competition with those staff members." (*Nurse-Midwifery Associates*, p. i)

On March 14, 1988, the U.S. District Court granted a partial summary judgment. The case was appealed to the United States Court of Appeals for the Sixth Circuit. On the question of intracorporate conspiracy between doctors and hospitals, the appeals court ruled that a hospital and the physicians on its staff are not sufficiently differentiated for intracorporate conspiracy to restrain trade to occur. The court looked differently at the interaction between physicians and SVMIC. The court ruled that there was the potential for physicians acting as individuals to conspire to unlawfully restrain competition among providers of maternity care by denying them malpractice insurance.

The case was appealed to the United States Supreme Court, but the Court refused to hear the case. There is some conflict among circuit courts on the question of whether a hospital and its medical staff are capable of conspiracy under the provisions of the Sherman Antitrust Act. While the Sixth Circuit Court ruled that in their view hospitals and doctors are not sufficiently differentiated for conspiracy to occur, another court might have ruled differently on this issue.

While the NMA case may have failed to meet the legal standard necessary for intracorporate conspiracy as interpreted by the Sixth Circuit Court of Appeals, what is clear in this case is the power of physicians in relation to nurse-midwives and even to other physicians who challenge the dominant model of childbirth. The power of physicians to block the plans of Sizemore and Henderson was manifested by their influence over the institutions within which they worked, their professional interaction with other institutions, and their role in shaping policy regarding insurance and in determining who would be insured and under what circumstances.

Sizemore and Henderson had to disband NMA and find work under different circumstances. They faced serious financial difficulties because they could not repay their bank loan due to the loss of their business. Eventually they did receive some money in settlement from some of the parties to the suit. Martin's obstetric practice in Nashville was ruined, and he was forced to start again in another location.

There have been similar cases involving nurse-midwives from other states, including California, New Jersey, and Missouri (Edwards and Waldorf, 1984,

p. 180; Sallomi, Pallow-Fleury, and McMahon, 1982). It is important to recognize that there is often a discrepancy between what nurse-midwives are allowed to do by law and what actually takes place. If the medical establishment refuses to cooperate with midwives, then midwives will not be able to function. Furthermore, in states where an alliance between physicians and nurse-midwives is required, the specific agreement between the physicians and the nurse-midwives determines what the nurse-midwives can do in their practice.

While the above discussion focuses on the conflict between physicians, on the one hand, and lay or nurse-midwives on the other, the conflict is more specifically between those who adhere to the medical model of childbirth and those who adhere to the midwifery model. Physicians who share the midwives' philosophy of birth as a healthy process requiring minimal intervention and who support out-of-hospital settings for birth are often subject to the same types of harassment experienced by midwives. The experience of Martin and his association with NMA demonstrates this point.

Another example is that of Dr. George Wootan, a family practitioner in Kingston, New York. Wootan had been attending home births for a number of years before disciplinary proceedings were brought against him by his colleagues in 1981. Dr. Wootan was accused of failing to diagnose a number of conditions including postpartum hemorrhage. His license to practice was suspended by the New York state health commissioner because his methods constituted an "imminent danger to the health of the people of New York State." While none of the charges specifically mentioned home birth, Wootan maintained that they all arose from that portion of his work. According to Wootan, his home birth practice cost the two area hospitals about $250,000 a year in lost revenue. The charge that Wootan had failed to recognize postpartum hemorrhage stemmed from a case involving a woman who was a Jehovah's Witness and who refused to go to the hospital because of her religious beliefs. Wootan said that he had, of course, recognized postpartum hemorrhage, but that he could not force an adult woman to go to a hospital against her will (Whitehouse, 1981).

CONSUMER INVOLVEMENT

Challenges to the medical model of childbirth came as early as the 1930s with the publication of Grantley Dick-Read's *Natural Childbirth* (Rothman, 1982). Read's work focused on preparing women for childbirth by eliminating fear. Doing so, Read believed, would eliminate pain.

In the 1950s, the work of Dr. Ferdinand Lamaze was introduced in the United States by Marjorie Karmel, who published *Thank You, Dr. Lamaze:*

A Mother's Experience in Painless Childbirth, after giving birth with Lamaze in Paris in 1955. The Lamaze method, Rothman argues, did not simply prepare women for childbirth. It prepared women for hospital birth. In 1960, Karmel founded the American Society for Psychoprophylaxis in Obstetrics (ASPO). ASPO has never challenged the basic structure of hospital birth. Instead its primary concern has been the use of anesthesia (Rothman, 1982, p. 90).

Since the beginning of the 1970s, however, there have been consumer movements in childbirth which pose a more direct challenge to the medical model. These movements can be traced at least in part to the larger women's health movement which began to develop in the late 1960s. Opposition to the medical control of birth, and support for midwifery and out-of-hospital birth, come from a variety of diverse sources. Within the home birth movement in the United States, for example, there is an alliance of feminist and traditionalist women and men. Feminists see childbirth as one component of the larger issue of reproductive rights. Women need to be able to have control over their bodies and their lives. The struggle over the conditions under which women will be pregnant, labor, and give birth are part of the larger struggle in which feminists are engaged. For those who identify as traditionalists, issues concerning childbirth are related to concerns regarding the family and the role of women as mothers (Rothman, 1982). Still other opponents of the medical model fall somewhere in between these two positions, maintaining that alternatives are safer and cheaper than hospital births and that they create competition for hospitals which will ultimately improve hospital care and services.

The ideological diversity among childbirth activists can lead to tensions and problems in determining political direction. While the medical profession is strongly unified in its support for the medical model, the other side is not nearly so organized in its support of the midwifery model. There is a clear divergence between feminists and traditionalists. There is a home birth movement which is supported by many but not all childbirth activists. There is a movement to support free-standing birth centers. Finally, there are some tensions among midwives themselves (Rothman, 1982; Martin, 1987).

At the same time that this diversity of views can be counterproductive, it is also encouraging to see women of diverse political perspectives uniting to change the conditions for women in childbirth. As Rothman states:

> The home-birth movement and midwifery strike a responsive chord in
> both feminist and strongly traditionalist women, because the underlying
> ideology is strongly woman-centered. The more traditional women are
> more comfortable when the woman is linked into a family structure,

and the more feminist women, when the woman is considered as an individual; but they share a view of the mother as having both the right and the ability to mother in her own way. At a time when one hears so much about the splintering of the women's movement, I find it heartening to see counterculture women from communities, suburban housewives, and feminist activists all organizing around a single issue. (Rothman, 1982, p. 110)

The work which childbirth activists do can take many forms. It can include the practice of lay midwifery; attempts to pass legislation favorable to midwives and out-of-hospital birth settings; support for midwives faced with legal difficulties; the establishment of out-of-hospital birth centers; and attempts to alter hospital policies on such matters as the presence of siblings at birth, the routine use of fetal heart monitoring, and the establishment of birthing rooms within the hospital setting.

DISCUSSION

Midwives, whether they are lay midwives, direct-entry midwives, or nurse-midwives, lack the professional autonomy necessary to direct their own practice and control their own profession. It may be that professional autonomy requires the demedicalization of childbirth. This, of course, is not easy to do because of the need for networking and backup services (Rothman, 1982, pp. 73–74).

Despite the differences among midwives, it is important to consider the overwhelmingly positive responses of women and families who seek the services of midwives. Eakins (1986b) found that women who gave birth out of hospital with a midwife, whether at home or in a free-standing birth center, expressed a high degree of satisfaction with their birth experiences.

In the course of my own research, I have interviewed women who have given birth at home as well as in a free-standing birth center. These women expressed highly positive feelings about their birth experiences and toward their midwives. Many of the women who gave birth at home had also reported extremely negative hospital experiences.

In the previous chapter, I included a quote from Lynn, who described her experience with a drunk physician who missed her birth and then, upon his arrival, tore her perineum with his bare hands. What follows is a quote from Lynn about the birth of her twins at home:

Here it was, my house and I could have those babies how I felt comfortable. And I felt like I could provide the best birth for them.

Whereas in the hospital I was at people's mercy . . . [at home] I got up, took a shower in my own bathroom and came back. They [the midwives] had changed the sheets, dressed the babies. It was wonderful. That morning was just one of the best mornings of my life. Just to snuggle with those babies, and the sun was coming up and it was just—it was wonderful. There's nothing to compare with it. It was just terrific.

This is how Julia described her labor at home, "It was a hard labor but I felt so supported and just whatever I wanted to help me through this they would do for me. Barbara [her labor support person] was massaging the balls of my feet, which I recommend to everyone I run into—it was wonderful. Rich [her husband] was rubbing my back, Karen [one of the midwives] was rubbing my legs. That really helped a lot."

Women who gave birth at the free-standing birth center I studied report similar experiences. They describe the support and encouragement they felt and the control they exercised over the circumstances of their births. Often these positive feelings apply even when a desired birth center experience ends with the birth taking place in a hospital. While the nurse-midwives from the birth center have no practicing privileges at either of the nearby hospitals, they do go along as support persons, often acting as a buffer between the birthing woman and the hospital staff. Many birth center clients form lasting relationships with their midwives as well as with the nurses who provide support and assistance at the center. Some clients become childbirth activists as a result of their birth experience.

Because of what midwifery has to offer, it is important that it be nurtured and sustained. Midwifery is not obstetrics. It offers us a different understanding of birth. It leads us to question long-held beliefs about the physiology of birth which come out of medical management, and it reminds us that birth is not only a physiological event. Birth is also an important event in the lives of women and families, and midwifery honors that fact. Midwifery offers us a view of birth which does not revolve around the concept of risk and is not rooted in fear. It offers theory and practice which are enriching and empowering for women.

As Rothman reminds us, "The demand by midwives to practice their profession is not an attempt by a less qualified group to engage in the practice of medicine, as it has most often been seen, but rather the claim of a more qualified group to practice midwifery" (Rothman, 1989, p. 183). Within the current structure nurse-midwives are defined as subordinate to doctors. Licensed direct-entry midwives often complain about state restrictions on their practice following licensure. DeVries (1985, p. 140) has argued that state sanction of midwives does not increase their autonomy.

Rather, it formalizes the power and control which physicians have over midwives.

As many midwives have pointed out, midwifery is an art as well as a science. It requires skills such as intuition and sensitivity as well as more technical and quantitative abilities. Seeing birth in nonmedical terms creates the possibility for autonomy for midwives as well as for the full recognition of what the theory and practice of midwifery have to offer.

5

Free-Standing Birth Centers

Free-standing birth centers (FSBCs)are nonhospital birthing facilities which are geographically and, usually, administratively separate from hospitals. It is important to distinguish free-standing birth centers from alternative birth centers (ABCs) which are in-hospital facilities which provide family-centered maternity care. Although ABCs may have a more homelike appearance than standard hospital labor and delivery facilities, all the high-tech equipment which has come to characterize hospital birth is at hand. Such equipment is hidden behind curtains or screens or in drawers, or it may be wheeled in as needed (Klee, 1986).

Primary care in free-standing birth centers is usually provided by nurse-midwives. The National Birth Center Study (Rooks et al., 1989) reported that certified nurse-midwives and students of nurse-midwifery provided the care during 78.6 percent of the labors and 80.6 percent of the births which occurred at the centers participating in the study. But birth centers are not always owned by nurse-midwives. In the summer of 1984 the National Association of Childbearing Centers (NACC) surveyed those birth centers known to them at the time. Questionnaires were mailed to 130 centers. Of these, 93 centers responded. Only 15 percent of the centers responding were owned by nurse-midwives alone. Physicians owned 32.2 percent. In a few cases centers were co-owned by nurse-midwives and physicians. Other centers were owned by a hospital, business group, community agency, or religious order (*NACC News*, fall/winter 1984–85). More recent research indicates that the trend toward physician ownership has continued and is increasing (Mathews and Zadak, 1991).

Care in birth centers reflects the assumptions that pregnant women are healthy as a rule and that pregnancy is a healthy process. Ideally birth takes place within the context of the family, and control rests with the family. There is a focus on prevention, of which education is an important part. When women have information about pregnancy they can care for themselves in ways which help to insure healthy outcomes. Ernst maintains that the model of care at birth centers is the midwifery model. Most nurse-midwives practicing in birth centers embrace the woman-centered approach which this model implies. Care is involved and intimate. Importance is attached to a close relationship between clients and caregivers, rooted in a sharing of information and mutual respect. There is a commitment on the part of caregivers that responsibility and control should rest with clients (Ernst, 1985).

At the same time that birth centers challenge the medical model, they are part of the system of health care delivery. Eunice Ernst, former executive director of the National Association of Childbearing Centers, has said that the birth center is "a first level of entry into an interdependent system for providing comprehensive care which requires providers to bring together their individual knowledge, skills, and services to form a unified whole" (Ernst, 1985). To this end nurse-midwives working in birth centers usually work in collaboration with physicians who provide consultation and backup. If complications arise during a birth which require a hospital transfer, a backup physician will take over in the hospital setting. In many cases, nurse-midwives can accompany their clients to the hospital and remain with them throughout the labor and birth.

Births at birth centers generally involve little intervention. Women are encouraged to labor at home until they are in active labor. Once they arrive at the centers in labor, they are encouraged and supported to give birth without painkilling medication or augmentation. Episiotomies are not done routinely. Most women continue to eat or drink during labor. Women can take showers or baths for relaxation. Most women at birth centers are accompanied by family and friends, often including other children, who are encouraged to be involved during labor and birth. Family and friends are also welcome at prenatal visits.

Although routine intervention is avoided at birth centers, birth center births involve more intervention than home births. In the 11,814 birth center births studied by Rooks et al. (1989) 1.3 percent involved artificial rupture of the membranes or oxytocin to induce labor. Intravenous infusions were used in 14.7 percent of the cases and 9.3 percent of the women in the sample had enemas. Twenty-four percent of women giving birth for the first time had an analgesic, tranquilizer, or sedative during labor, compared with 6.2 percent of the women who had had one or more previous births. Vacuum extraction was used in 0.4 percent of the births and forceps in 0.2 percent. Episiotomies were done in 17.6 percent of the cases.

Women seeking care in an FSBC must be judged to be at low risk for obstetrical complications. The criteria for judging risk are generally the same as those used by obstetricians. Birth center care is provided in a comfortable, homelike atmosphere. Centers differ quite a bit one from the next, but they share some similarities. The birthing rooms look like bedrooms which might be found in a typical home. Many birth centers have other rooms which can be used by birthing women, their families, and friends. There might be a kitchen for preparing meals or snacks, a place for watching TV, and spaces where children can play. The birth center which I studied has, among other amenities, a Jacuzzi which can be used for relaxation during labor.

BIRTH CENTERS AND THE MEDICAL MODEL: ISSUES OF POWER AND CONTROL

The first birth centers were formed to serve rural populations. In 1975, the Maternity Center Association of New York City (MCA) established the first free-standing birth center in an urban area (Rooks et al., 1989). The initiative to do so came from a new determination in some childbearing couples to stay out of the hospital for birth. According to Lubic (1981), these families needed three things from their childbirth experience— safety, satisfaction, and economy—which the medical model was not supplying. The Maternity Center Association had four possible options in trying to meet the needs of disaffected childbearing couples: (1) try to humanize the hospital setting; (2) establish a free-standing, full-scale maternity hospital; (3) return to a home birth system similar to one which they had operated from 1931 to 1959; or (4) open a free-standing birth center.

They chose the last option, believing that it best met the three criteria. In January 1974, MCA's board of directors filed an application with the state of New York for permission to establish a center. MCA was required to demonstrate both the need for and the feasibility of the project they were proposing. They were expected to provide evidence of the qualifications of future staff along with backup letters of support from obstetricians, pediatricians, and public health physicians. The model for the center was the home, not the hospital. Care was to be provided by a team consisting of obstetricians, nurse-midwives, pediatricians, and public health nurses. Client families would be directly involved in decision making. Four nearby hospitals agreed to provide emergency backup, and the Visiting Nurse Service of New York agreed to do follow-up home visits.

There was, of course, opposition to the project from some members of the medical community, particularly obstetricians and pediatricians. A well-known neonatologist suggested that those involved with the project would "kill babies" (Lubic, 1981, p. 232). There were meetings held to answer criticisms launched by the medical community, including the following objections: (1) that the MCA birth center would be too far from a hospital to be safe (the closest backup hospital was seven blocks away) and (2) that the MCA staff would be unable to define "normal" in a way that would avoid risk to babies. One recommendation which came out of the discussion was that MCA should try to formalize backup arrangements with one hospital rather than four.

There were some minor confrontations with the city of New York and some difficulties over third-party reimbursement, but the MCA Childbearing Center did open in September 1975. Some problems continued after the center's opening. The state notified MCA that it required a formal written agreement with the backup hospital. When the center opened in 1975, they had four such agreements. In June 1976, MCA received word from one of their backup hospitals that they were canceling the agreement because they were going to become self-insured. Several months later another backup institution canceled the arrangement, citing disapproval of the project by the obstetrical profession as the reason. A short time later, the health department began to insist on an updated formal agreement and one of the original four hospitals did agree to update its arrangement. Other problems soon surfaced. One of the backup physicians was told that he would have his hospital admitting privileges revoked if he continued his work with the Childbearing Center.

While the MCA Childbearing Center was established and continues to operate, some of the same problems which plagued Nurse-Midwifery Associates were also evident here. Problems with physician backup and institutional support were most critical. MCA was able to work out arrangements which made it possible for them to remain in operation, but as the Nurse-Midwifery Associates case demonstrates, that is not always possible.

Lubic (1981) argues that childbearing centers threaten both medical control and the fee-for-service model of health care. Interestingly, however, Lubic also argues that childbearing centers also pose a threat to some nurse-midwives who have been practicing in a hospital setting and have become dependent upon physicians and hospital-based technology. Such centers also threaten those nurse-midwives who emulate the economic aspects of the medical model and whose primary goal is making more money. For them, the salary structure of birth centers may be unacceptable. Lubic states: "In our experience and opinion midwifery in CbC [childbearing centers] offers satisfactions which cannot be approached in the hospital setting. Essential to the viability of such centers will be the nurse-midwife's understanding that the costs of normal childbirth must be reduced and the extraordinary monetary rewards of physician specialists cannot be considered an approachable standard" (Lubic, 1981, p. 245).

According to Lubic, the only way to avoid high-tech obstetrics is to remove birth from the hospital setting. Despite strong opposition MCA did establish a low-cost facility where nurse-midwives can practice free of the constraints which hospitals impose (Edwards and Waldorf, 1984, pp.183–185). Since 1975, at least 240 other birth centers have opened in the United States, although many of these have since closed, primarily as a result of the malpractice insurance crisis (Rooks et al., 1989). As of 1995, NACC in conjunction with the ACNM, an insurance administrator, and insurance companies, have put together an insurance package specifically for birth centers. The package covers all members of the birth center staff including nurses, nurse-midwives, and consulting physicians. At present, part-time staff members are not covered by the package but such coverage may be available in the future.

Rothman (1989, 1983, 1982) has argued that when nurse-midwives work in the physician-controlled environment of the hospital, they are not free to develop their own knowledge or to train incoming nurse-midwives according to their own standards and criteria. Professional autonomy for nurse-midwives may require that they opt out of the medical system. As pointed out earlier, however, this is not easy to do. Nurse-midwives are dependent upon physicians for backup services. Ideally, the relationship between nurse-midwives and their backup physicians is trusting and collegial, but this is not always the case. This is particularly a problem for nurse-midwives who attend home births.

Attending home births also presents some other problems for nurse-midwives. Physician backup is sometimes difficult to come by. Often nurse-midwives are not permitted to accompany home birth clients to the hospital when a transfer occurs. Nurse-midwives who provide home birth services find themselves on call most of the time. If they practice alone they have the constant worry about what to do if two clients go into labor at the same time. The time demands of a home birth practice make it necessary to limit the number of one's clients. This, in turn, means that it is sometimes difficult to support oneself on the income from a home-birth practice (Rothman, 1983).

Free-standing birth centers can provide a compromise for nurse-midwives between the hospital environment and a home-based practice. Free-standing birth centers may provide as ideal a work setting for nurse-midwives as they are likely to find (Rothman, 1983). Centers can provide for nurse-midwives the advantages which hospitals provide for practitioners. In birth centers, for example, there is often a shared responsibility with other nurse-midwives. This is, of course, dependent upon how many nurse-midwives are on staff. It is typically the case that nurse-midwives practicing in birth centers have an agreement with a physician or physicians who will provide consultation and backup services. Within the setting of the birth center, nurse-midwives are usually free from the legal vulnerability which often plagues home birth practitioners.

Birth centers also usually provide nurse-midwives with a high degree of professional autonomy to make decisions and set policy. It is important to note, however, that the degree of autonomy over policy depends upon the kind of administrative relationship which birth centers have with hospitals. Annandale (1988), for example, writes about nurse-midwives practicing in a birth center licensed through an adjacent hospital. Although Annandale characterizes this birth center as free-standing, the administrative connection to the hospital gives the hospital a great deal of control over the practice of the nurse-midwives at the center. Annandale's study demonstrates this point. During the first four years of operation at the center, there were no formal restrictions put on the timing of labor or on when a backup obstetrician should be consulted. In the middle of the fourth year, however, new protocols were introduced which required (1) that pelvic examinations be done every three hours once a woman was in active labor and (2) that a physician be called if a woman had been pushing for two hours, if she had been fully dilated for two hours, or if she was in active labor and had made no progress for three hours. The changes were made as a result of pressure from the hospital administration and obstetricians.

Annandale (1988) argues that nurse-midwifery practice in a free-standing birth center actually represents an interaction between the medical and midwifery models. The midwives Annandale studied saw birth as an instinctual process. Birthing women were encouraged to follow their "natural instincts" and "take responsibility" for the birth. Women were expected to be active participants in their own care. At prenatal visits they were expected to weigh themselves and do their own urinalysis and then enter this data on their medical charts. There was also the stated expectation that women could "run their own labor" (Annandale, 1988, p. 96). However, pressure from obstetricians that births conform to particular patterns and standards often ran directly contrary to the values of the nurse-midwives. In addition, they found that in many cases they had led women to expect a "patient-directed" birth which they could not provide. Nurse-midwives often found themselves in the position of having to balance obstetrical authority and demands, the hopes and anxieties of clients, and their own birth ideology. At the same time that these nurse-midwives were trying to provide an alternative to the medical model, they found themselves engaged in it.

Maurin (1980) also demonstrates the problems associated with trying to negotiate an out-of-hospital birthing service within a structural context of medical control. Maurin studied a free-standing birth center, Western Birth Center, which opened in 1975. She identifies some of the same problems which MCA experienced, and she stresses the power of the gatekeeping position which physicians occupy with regard to gaining access to needed services and resources. Initially, a physician was appointed as medical director of Western Birth Center. He was not an obstetrician and, at the time of his appointment, he was in a full-time residency program. Having very little direct involvement with the center, he served mainly "as a figurehead whose signature was valuable on occasion" (Maurin, 1980, p. 321). At the end of his residency, he decided to try to establish himself as the person in charge at the center. The nurse-midwife who had been acting in that capacity chal-lenged him. It was she who was, in fact, providing the services which clients were seeking and, beyond this, she owned the building in which the center was housed. During this conflict, the medical director asked the board of directors to fire the nurse-midwife. She, in turn, threatened not to renew the lease on the building. In the end, the medical director resigned, and the board of directors eliminated his position.

The resignation proved costly to the birth center because they lost their insurance reimbursement as a result. While serving as medical director, the physician had negotiated for third-party reimbursement for a portion of the services provided by the center. Since services were not being provided in a hospital, the insurance company would not pay the institutional fee. They did agree to pay the professional fee as long as there was a physician's signature on the insurance forms. Once the insurance company learned of the director's resignation, they informed Western Birth Center that they would no longer honor claims from the center. It was their policy only to reimburse physician services. The nurse-midwife tried to explain that services at the center had never been provided by physicians but was unable to convince the insurance company to resume reimbursement to anyone but a physician.

While the nurse-midwives at Western Birth Center experienced many setbacks, they were able to keep the center going. Maurin credits the success of the birth center to the ability of nurse-midwives to negotiate arrangements with individual physicians which allowed official rules to be circumvented. It was the nurse-midwives who actually provided all the care for birthing women who came to the center, yet they did so in a way that left the power of physicians intact. As Maurin notes, "When these actions are performed by a non-physician, however, they are done within the context of a negotiated relationship between physician and non-physician whereby one party is persuaded or manipulated to consent to the exception. At this level of negotiation in the workplace almost anything is negotiable, but the institutionalized role definitions remain unchanged. Thus, while permitting exceptions, these negotiations protect and preserve the overall structure" (Maurin, 1980, p. 328). As Maurin points out, to actually change institutionalized roles means changing power relations. In the case of Western Birth Center, negotiated arrangements made it possible for services to be provided at the same time that the overall power structure was left unchanged, contributing to the vulnerability of the birth center.

Annandale and Maurin identify the crux of the problems faced by birth centers. They attempt to offer a nonhospital alternative to the physician-controlled medical model at the same time that they are defined and constrained by this model.

Rothman (1983) argues that while free-standing birth centers often meet the needs of nurse-midwives as a work environment, they do not necessarily meet the needs of clients, particularly those who "see birth as a fully normal and healthy occurrence and want to integrate birth into family life" (1983, p. 7). Rothman argues that as an alternative to home birth, birth centers have some disadvantages. They require travel both during labor and shortly following birth. While birth centers may be pleasant and comfortable and look "like home," they are not home. Free-standing birth centers appear safer than hospitals, but there is no evidence that they are safer than the home as an environment for birth.

It is important to consider that FSBCs have a cultural advantage over home birth. Most people in our society view birth as requiring hospitalization, and very few choose home birth. While there may be no scientific evidence supporting the choice of hospital over home, the cultural beliefs surrounding birth make it very difficult to reject the medical model of birth. Some women who would not consider home birth are willing to consider birthing at an FSBC. Free-standing birth centers do challenge the medical model and they do provide an environment where birthing women can experience much more power over birth than a hospital experience would allow. Birth center clients who express satisfaction with their birth center experiences express a greater willingness to consider a home birth for subsequent births. Rothman (1983, p. 7) suggests that this can be viewed as a success on the part of birth centers in "resocializing their clients to think of birth in non-medical ways."

It is true that birth centers are not home, but they are vastly different from hospitals. The atmosphere is homelike, not institutional. The philosophy which guides the practice of nurse-midwives practicing in birth centers is one which sees birth as a healthy process. When women enter hospitals to give birth, they may be going to a place they have never been to before. If they have been there before, it may have been to visit a patient or maybe to take a tour offered to prospective parents who are planning a birth at the hospital. Women who go to birth centers to give birth are going to a place which is familiar to them, where they will be cared for by people (nurse-midwives, nurses, sometimes doctors) who are familiar to them. They will have gone to the birth center for their prenatal care. They may have attended prenatal classes and childbirth classes at the center. Centers also sometimes host social events, public lectures and workshops, and classes for prospective and new parents. Many women who have gone to birth centers describe very warm feelings for the place as well as the people at the centers.

STATISTICAL DATA: THE NATIONAL BIRTH CENTER STUDY

Both statistical and anecdotal evidence indicates a high degree of client satisfaction with birth centers. Rooks et al. (1989) studied 11,814 birth center clients. Among those women who were not transferred to the hospital during labor, 75.7 percent completed evaluations of their experience. Of this number, 98.8 percent said that they would recommend the birth center to friends, and 94 percent said that they would use the birth center again. Of the women who were transferred to a hospital, 54.1 percent completed evaluations. Of these, 96.9 percent said they would recommend the center to friends, while 83.3 percent said they would use the center again. Eakins (1986b) reports that 87 percent of the women in her study who gave birth in free-standing birth centers were positive or extremely positive about their births. Eakins argues that for women giving birth in FSBCs as well as at home, the psychological outcome was very positive. She attributes this to the ability to control the birth situation which exists for women in out-of-hospital settings.

In the study done by Rooks et al., the authors compared the characteristics of birth center clients with those of the general population of childbearing women. They looked at the incidence of complications in birth centers along with the rate of hospital transfer, and finally, they discussed general outcomes for women who gave birth in birth centers and their newborns.

In comparing the characteristics of women admitted to birth centers in labor between 1985 and 1987 with those of all U.S. women who gave birth in 1986, the study found many similarities as well as some interesting differences. In both groups the vast majority of women giving birth fell between the ages of eighteen and thirty-four. Among the birth center population, 89.9 percent of women fell into this category as opposed to 88.3 percent among the general population of women giving birth. Only 2.3

percent of women giving birth in birth centers were under eighteen years old, as compared with 4.7 percent of all U.S. women who gave birth in 1986.

Women giving birth in birth centers had more education overall than the general population. Of those giving birth in birth centers, 12.4 percent had less than twelve years of education, compared with 15.5 percent of U.S. women who gave birth in 1986. Among birth center clients 32.3 percent had twelve years of schooling, compared with 43.7 percent of the larger group. The number of birth center clients who had between thirteen and fifteen years of education was 23.5 percent, compared with 22.1 percent for the general population. There was a much higher percentage of women in the birth center group with sixteen or more years of education (31.8 percent) than in the general population of U.S. women giving birth in 1986 (18.7 percent).

There were some striking racial differences between these two groups. While 16.5 percent of U.S. women who gave birth in 1986 were black, only 3.9 percent of the birth center population was black. Hispanic women, on the other hand, made up 16.3 percent of the birth center clientele and 11.0 percent of the more general population of women giving birth. It is important to point out, however, that four birth centers accounted for more than 80 percent of the Hispanic women in the sample. Non-Hispanic white women accounted for 78.4 percent of the birth center women and 68.1 percent of U.S. women giving birth in 1986.

Birth center clients were less likely to begin prenatal care in the first trimester (61.7 percent) compared with the larger group (75.9 percent), but birth center clients were also less likely not to receive any prenatal care or to have care delayed until the third trimester (3.4 percent), compared with the larger population of women giving birth (6.0 percent).

Birth center clients were less likely to smoke or drink alcohol during pregnancy. They were less likely to be unmarried and slightly less likely to be poor than the general population of women. Birth center clients were less likely to give birth before thirty-seven weeks of gestation (2.4 percent) than the larger group (10.0 percent), and they were less likely to give birth to a baby with a birthweight of less than 2,501 grams (0.8 percent) than the more general population (6.8 percent) (Rooks et al., pp. 1805–1806). The authors are careful to point out, however, that most birth center clients who had preterm labor or who experienced intrauterine growth retardation were transferred to the hospital and as a result were not included in the study results. These outcomes, then, cannot be attributed to prenatal care received at birth centers.

One concern which is frequently raised about birth centers has to do with their safety in comparison to hospitals. This concern is rooted in a belief in the technocratic approach to birth, which assumes that the high-tech environment of the hospital offers the safest environment for birth. Since it is a widely held cultural belief that hospitals provide the safest environment, evidence which would support this belief is rarely requested. It is widely assumed that out-of-hospital settings are less safe, so it is important to be able to demonstrate empirically that this is not the case.

Of the 11,814 women admitted to birth centers in labor, 15.8 percent were transferred to hospitals during labor or shortly after birth. Of the 15.8 percent who were transferred to hospitals, only 2.4 percent were emergency transfers. The Cesarean section rate was 4.4 percent and there were no maternal deaths. Of the women who birthed at the birth centers, 99.4 percent had spontaneous vaginal deliveries. Twenty percent of women and their newborns experienced no complications at all during labor, birth, or immediately following birth. Another group, representing 50.8 percent of the birth center sample, had complications which were neither life threatening nor likely to cause permanent damage (including transient fetal distress, failure to progress, and less than fourth-degree perineal lacerations). In 21.3 percent of the women there were somewhat more serious complications (including moderate shoulder dystocia, retained placenta, and hypertension). Serious emergency complications occurred in 7.9 percent of birth center cases, with 47.1 percent of those women being transferred to a hospital.

Women who had borne no previous children were most likely to be transferred to hospitals. The transfer rate for this group of women or their infants was 28.9 percent, compared with only 7.3 percent of women who had borne previous children.

Rooks et al. used Apgar scores and mortality rates as final outcome measures in their study. Apgar scores rate an infant's condition immediately following birth. The score represents an evaluation of the infant's heart rate, respiratory effort, muscle tone, reflex irritability, and color. The infant is given a score on each of the five criteria ranging from 0 (low) to 2 (normal); evaluations are performed at one minute and at five minutes after birth. It is typical for the five-minute score to be higher than the one-minute score. A low total score (0 to 3) is an indication of serious distress, moderate distress is indicated by a score of 4 to 7, and a score of 8 to10 indicates that the infant is doing well (Bernstein, 1993, p. 278). Among the babies in the study, 0.6 percent had five-minute Apgar scores of below 7. There were 11,826 births to the 11,814 mothers in the study and fifteen intrapartum or neonatal deaths. Of the deaths, seven were due to lethal congenital abnormalities. The stillbirth rate was 0.4 per 1,000 births, and the neonatal mortality rate was 0.8 per 1,000 births. There were no maternal deaths.

The study done by Rooks et al. is a descriptive study. They did not have a control sample of hospital births for comparison. The authors, however, do compare the birth center outcomes with data from five studies of low-risk hospital births. The incidences of low Apgar scores and mortality rates among infants in the birth center sample were in the same range as in the hospital studies. The Cesarean section rate among birth center clients was roughly half that among low-risk hospital women in the two studies which reported these rates. It is important to note that the hospital data spanned the years 1969 to 1985. Over that period of time, rates of Cesarean sections in hospitals have increased dramatically. If the birth center Cesarean section rate of 4.4 percent was compared with more recent hospital data, it is likely that the difference in the rate would be even more dramatic.

The data presented by Rooks et al. demonstrate that birth centers have good outcomes and a low rate of Cesarean sections. It is important to remember that these births occur, for the most part, without the use of invasive procedures. Rooks et al. also point out that birth center services are less expensive than hospital services. Birth centers usually charge about half of what hospitals charge for a routine vaginal birth. Birth centers are small and nonbureaucratic and can be designed to meet the needs of particular populations and communities. Some birth centers are located in rural areas, serving populations too small to support a hospital obstetric service. Others serve urban populations. Within the last few years the Maternity Center Association of New York opened a birth center in the Morris Heights section of the South Bronx. A video entitled *Hope Reborn* documents some of the effects which this birth center has had on the women in that community. Women who have come to the center during pregnancy and birth have received quality care and had good birth outcomes. But the effects of care which empowers women extend way beyond the birth experience. Women, and even their partners, see themselves differently as a result of their birth center experience. They feel empowered in other areas of their lives, including parenting and work, and they express pride in themselves and their community.

DISCUSSION

Free-standing birth centers are an important option for birthing women and their families. They offer an out-of-hospital location for birth which is nurturing and supportive. Nurse-midwives in free-standing birth facilities usually practice according to the midwifery model, offering intimate, involved care to women and families.

Birth is not viewed narrowly as a medical event. Rather, it is seen as an important event which changes the lives of all the participants—family members, friends, and even the nurse-midwives themselves. As the Morris

Heights example demonstrates, the empowerment that comes from the kinds of positive birth experiences which birth centers facilitate can extend far beyond birth and parenting. It can extend to the workplace and to the community at large.

As many of the examples in this chapter show, however, birth centers challenge the medical model at the same time that they are to some extent defined and constrained by it. The case study which follows discusses the establishment and operation of a free-standing birth center. It presents the important birthing option which the birth center brings to the community in which it is located. It also discusses the difficulties which the birth center has faced over its years of operation and which result mainly from its ambiguous location and status. The center poses a challenge to the medical model but is dependent upon established medical-legal interests for physician and hospital backup, for third-party reimbursement, and for malpractice insurance.

6

Case Study:
The Founding of a
Free-Standing Birth Center

In earlier chapters I have presented contrasting approaches to birth. I have maintained that nontechnocratic, woman-centered approaches such as the midwifery model empower women by valuing their knowledge, their experience, and their fully conscious participation in birthing their babies. In this chapter, I describe the formation of a free-standing birth center run by nurse-midwives. As the chapter shows, the reality of creating this type of out-of-hospital facility is complex and contradictory. Perhaps most important, the birth center was created in a legal, professional, political, and cultural environment dominated by medical and hospital elites. To some degree, the birth center is an accommodation to legal and medical authority. Despite these limits, it constitutes a location where women can assert their knowledge and responsibility in birthing.

THE SETTING

The state where I have been studying birthing practices is characterized by ambiguity and contradictions. On the one hand, there are a number of forces which oppose challenges to the medical model of birth. Traditional patterns of medical authority have been maintained. There is a strong core among the medical profession in the area which is vocally opposed to innovative medical facilities that challenge and disperse medical authority, such as out-of-hospital surgical centers and birth centers. They have also opposed broadening the practice of nonphysician practitioners such as nurse-anesthetists, nurse-practitioners, and nurse-midwives. The local medical center has a virtual monopoly over the provision of hospital services in the area. Its only competition comes from two small hospitals. As a result there is very limited pressure to respond to consumer demands. Moreover, the local medical center is one of the largest employers in the area. In the past it has discouraged its own employees from using facilities such as birth centers by denying reimbursement for such facilities in its health insurance policies. Nurses in the area have been working to establish greater autonomy from physicians both inside and outside of the hospital setting, but with only limited success. Under state law, lay midwifery is illegal except in rare circumstances. The practice of nurse-midwifery is allowed provided that practicing nurse-midwives can provide written evidence that they are working in collaboration with a physician. Under the Advanced Practice Nursing Act passed in 1994, nurse-midwives and other advanced practice nurses have the authority to write prescriptions.

On the other hand, there are a number of forces that are open to changes in the provision of medical services. Despite the generally conservative climate, the birth center concept is supported by one of the largest and most popular obstetric practices in the area. Within the birth center's first year of operation, most of the major organizations and institutions that contract with Blue Cross/Blue Shield designated the birth center for reimbursement. Nurse-midwives and a committed group of consumers have consistently supported the availability of birth center services. Finally, the state health council, which was composed of a variety of health professionals and laypersons engaged in health planning for the state during the time that the birth center was being formed, was an important source of support for the birth center.

The response of the local medical center to the birth center project can be characterized as ambiguous at best. Anne Watson, the nurse-midwife who is currently director of the birth center, was formerly a director of parent education at the medical center. A conflict among Anne, the physicians, and the hospital administrators over comments Anne made to a reporter led to her dismissal from her position. This set the wheels in motion for the establishment of an out-of-hospital alternative to the obstetric services provided by the medical center. The medical center administration has never been and is not currently supportive of the practice of nurse-midwifery. Nurse-midwives do not have practicing privileges at the medical center. A high-ranking hospital administrator has been extremely critical of women who seek alternatives to dominant childbirth practices, referring to such women as "kooks" and "raving lunatics."

Yet since the birth center has been in operation, there have been no major conflicts between it and the medical center. The two places have a written agreement stating that the medical center will admit transfer clients from the birth center. Such an agreement assures that any necessary transfers are routinely carried out. In addition, the medical center sells supplies to the birth center. Since the medical center purchases supplies in such large quantity, they pay a much lower price for them than the birth center would have to pay when ordering in small quantities. The relationship between these two institutions, then, can be characterized as professional, but at the same time their philosophies toward childbirth are very different.

Local health planning agencies served as a source of support for the birth center project. The development of alternative obstetrical services was consistent with the goals of the state health plan for 1980–1985, which stressed the need for alternatives which were cost-effective and which met the varied needs of area consumers. The health council provided an important buffer between those trying to establish a birth center in the area and the many physicians trying to block the development of an out-of-hospital birthing facility.

Birth centers, like many contemporary health care facilities in the United States, are usually privately funded. The individuals or groups who try to establish birth centers must either have the necessary money themselves or have access to funds. Some states require that they be able to demonstrate financial stability. In this case, for example, the state required that before any person or group could file a certificate of need for a birth center, they had to have property or an option to buy property for the center. They also required that a birth center have twenty-five thousand dollars in cash or assets prior to opening. Financial considerations, then, were crucial in the efforts to establish a birth center in the state.

Support from sources beyond the individuals or groups involved in a project is always an important factor, but this is particularly true when the project is one which conflicts with established beliefs and practices. Support for birth centers often comes from the feminist community, from consumer advocates, from some health professionals, and from community groups. While there is an active and visible feminist community in the state which I studied, it did not play any significant role in the efforts to establish a birth center in the state. Consumer advocates, particularly Childbirth and Parenting Education Associates (CPEA), were somewhat involved in the birth center project, as were some local health professionals. The American College of Nurse-Midwives and the Cooperative Birth Center Network (now the National Association of Childbearing Centers) provided support from outside the state.

All of the elements discussed above are important features of the environment in which the efforts to establish a birth center took place and in which this center now operates. What follows is a discussion of the process by which the birth center was established. This discussion focuses on the important participants and events which were part of the process, including the different attempts by two groups to open a free-standing birth center. It elaborates upon the ways in which features of the operating environment enabled one group to succeed in their efforts while the other failed and in which those features shaped the conditions under which the birth center currently operates.

BABYPLACE

In the summer of 1980, a group of consumers, four women and one man, began working to open a birth center. I will refer to them and their proposed center as "Babyplace." All of the members of Babyplace had been active in childbirth issues in the area prior to their efforts to open a birth center. One of the members had been instrumental in getting the medical center to allow fathers to be present for Cesarean births. They hoped that Babyplace would open in 1982. Their initial concerns were raising money, gaining nonprofit status, and filing a certificate of need with the state health council. Even after these tasks were accomplished, however, it would be necessary for this group to find a nurse-midwife willing to provide prenatal care and attend births at the center. Since state law requires nurse-midwives to practice in alliance with a physician, they would have to locate a physician or group of physicians willing to enter into such an arrangement.

Babyplace began with serious financial problems and no significant base of support. The state bureau of health planning required anyone trying to establish a birth center to file a certificate of need in order to determine whether the proposed service was in line with the needs of consumers in the area and consistent with the goals of the health plan for the state. The group lacked the information necessary to fill out the application since they had no previous financial experience with birth centers and no projections on the number of births expected. In order to file, they also needed to own property or to have an option on property, but their lack of funds made acquiring property difficult.

The group incorporated quickly. They organized themselves hierarchically with each of the five active members of the group holding office as president, vice president, secretary, treasurer, and public relations director. In an effort to gain support for their project, Babyplace held a meeting at the local academy of medicine in October 1980, for area obstetricians, pediatricians, hospital administrators, and childbirth educators. The purpose of the meeting was to acquaint these childbirth "experts" with the plan which Babyplace had to open a free-standing birth center run by nurse-midwives. The speakers at the meeting were a nationally known neonatalogist and a certified nurse-midwife who was director of a family health service in a nearby state.

Both the doctor and the nurse-midwife spoke enthusiastically about birth centers and argued that they are preferable for low-risk mothers and their babies. The nurse-midwife reported that about 20 percent of her clients were from the area in which Babyplace was trying to establish a birth center. They were willing to make the one-hour drive to her center in order to have the type of birth experience that nurse-midwives and birth centers provide. The doctor argued that hospitals are not without risks and that there is a much lower incidence of infection for newborns at birth centers than in hospitals.

Attendance at the meeting was very small. Only three obstetricians out of over fifty who practice in the area attended the meeting. There were administrators present from both the local medical center and one of the smaller hospitals. A few childbirth educators and area pediatricians were also in attendance. The meeting was not open to the public, and there was no consumer representation. While the purpose of the meeting was to inform those present of the benefits of birth centers, the response from the audience indicated that they were not convinced. There were some perfunctory questions and very little discussion.

The meeting demonstrated the pronounced lack of interest in birth centers and nurse-midwifery on the part of medical experts in the area. Despite this meeting, the officers of Babyplace continued with their plans to open a birth center. As of January 1981, the group still had no money with which to purchase property. Their plan at that point was to apply for a grant which would be used toward the purchase of a building, although they had no clear idea where or how to apply for such funding. In addition, they sent out a letter to potential supporters requesting donations, along with a fact sheet explaining the Babyplace philosophy and a description of the services they intended to provide. The following are excerpts from the fact sheet:

What is the purpose of Babyplace, Inc.?

Babyplace, Inc., a nonprofit, tax-exempt group, will offer the woman and her family a choice of safe alternatives for childbearing. There are a growing number of couples who want more control over the births of their children. Babyplace proposes to meet these needs by combining the comfort of a home delivery with the security of professional guidance in close proximity to a hospital.

What is the philosophy of Babyplace, Inc.?

Childbearing is a natural process that must be treated with respect. Babyplace recognizes each woman and her family as unique individuals with their own set of values, feelings, choices, and medical needs.

Babyplace acknowledges that the newborn is a complete person with a unique personality that also must be respected.

Who is eligible to deliver at Babyplace, Inc.?

Any woman is eligible if she meets the medical criteria for low-risk mothers. The program at Babyplace will be designed to incorporate the family in the childbirth experience. The mother's progress will be closely followed by the nurse-midwives and obstetricians, with the parents taking equal responsibility for their own health maintenance.

The services which Babyplace intended to offer included counseling, child-birth education, prenatal care, nurse-midwife-attended birth, postpartum follow-up, breastfeeding counseling, parenting support, and education.

Babyplace had serious problems locating health professionals willing to work with them. A nurse-midwife from out of state agreed to work with Babyplace while they were becoming established, but a full-time nurse-mid-wife had to be found who could work on a permanent basis. Babyplace could not, however, hire a nurse-midwife when they had no money and no building and had not completed a certificate of need application. In the meantime, Babyplace was trying to locate an obstetrician who would provide backup support for the center. They had been turned down by all of the physicians whom they had approached.

At the same time that Babyplace was facing those obstacles, they learned that Anne Watson was considering filing a certificate of need to open a birth center in the area. Although they realized that this could create yet another obstacle for them, they decided to proceed independently with their plans.

By February 1981, Babyplace had established a board of directors which included a nurse-midwife, a minister, a counselor, and an attorney. The attorney served as an important source of advice, because legal questions regarding zoning, public health regulations, and midwifery law arose con-stantly. Despite the support of a board of directors, however, Babyplace still had no money and no backup support from physicians.

It was becoming clear to the Babyplace officers that they needed more exposure to and support from the community, but they seemed unclear about how to locate groups in the area that might back them and about how to generate their support. Their attorney suggested that because the opening of a birth center was a feminist issue, the feminist community was an important potential ally, but the Babyplace officers disagreed.

Some of the people involved in establishing Babyplace were keeping a close watch on the activities of Anne Watson, who had begun work to establish a birth center. They saw themselves in direct conflict with her and even discussed ways of undermining her efforts despite the advice of their attorney, who felt they should try to form an alliance. Anne was well known in the community and over the years had had conflicts with some local physicians and hospital administrators. As a way of keeping her from succeeding, the officers of Babyplace considered informing a local hospital administrator of her plans, so that he would put pressure on the physicians who were most likely to form an alliance with her to withdraw their support from the project.

Despite their opposition to Anne Watson's efforts, Babyplace did meet with her and the head of her board of directors in early March 1981 to discuss their respective plans. Prior to Anne's attempt to open a birth center in this area, she had been the director of midwifery services at a birth center in another state. She was well aware not only of the legal battles and the financial difficulties which opening any birth center entails, but also of the major stumbling blocks in this particular area. The primary problem was the monopoly of the medical center. The second problem was the legal requirement of physician backup for nurse-midwives. The two problems were clearly related: if the hospital administration and the majority of doctors were opposed to birth centers and nurse-midwives, they could bring administrative and peer pressure to bear on other physicians not to provide support for such practice. Lack of physician backup could effectively keep nurse-midwives from practicing. While money was a problem for both groups, Anne had access to enough capital to start a center. Both she and her board of directors clearly recognized the need for broad-based community support.

There was some discussion about whether the two groups might work together to open a center. Anne said cooperation was possible since the ultimate goal of the groups was the same, but that it was necessary to agree on a strategy for reaching that goal. She had a number of objections to Babyplace. She argued that the name was a bad choice because there was money to be made by providing well-woman care. Anne realized that free-standing birth centers are often financially marginal operations. Providing a range of services, including well-woman care, could be important to clients and could help to insure the financial stability of the birth center. People would not realize that a center known as Babyplace would provide anything but care related to pregnancy and birth. She also felt very strongly that a nurse-midwife must be the director of a birth center. While there could and should be consumers on the board of directors, it was important that the person in charge have the medical training and credentials necessary to make important decisions for the center. Finally, she felt that the Babyplace organization was administratively top heavy with five officers, none of whom had any medical credentials. The criticisms leveled against Babyplace by Anne made it clear that the only thing the two groups agreed upon was the ultimate goal of seeing a birth center open in the area. Their strategies on how to achieve that goal and how to organize the institutional structure of the center were very much at odds.

Anne's concerns about having people with medical credentials visible in the organization and about insuring financial stability stood in stark contrast to the efforts of Babyplace. After Anne left the March 1981 meeting, the officers of Babyplace discussed the idea of cooperation between the two groups. They agreed that they should not rush to join forces. They felt that the priorities of the two groups were different, although theirs were not made explicit. Also, the Babyplace officers were opposed to having a nurse-midwife as director of the center. Finally, the members were extremely critical of the nurse-midwife on a personal level. They expressed dislike for her as well as for those working with her.

The officers of Babyplace met again at the end of March 1981, but made no further progress toward establishing a birth center. There was a great deal of discussion about how to overcome zoning obstacles, but zoning was the least of their problems at this point. They still had no physician backup, and they were in agreement that no alliance with Anne was possible. In addition, the group discovered that the letter and fact sheet they had sent out in January had offended local childbirth educators and nursing mothers groups. Among the services that Babyplace said they would provide were childbirth education and breastfeeding counseling. Nursing mothers groups and childbirth educators felt that Babyplace intended to take over in these two areas and were upset by the infringement upon their areas of competence.

At this point, what little organization Babyplace had began to crumble. They still had no money, no physician backup, and no public support. Furthermore, they had no clear idea of how to generate such support. They offended groups that were obvious potential sources of it, they rejected the notion that birth centers were a feminist concern, and they had made no appeal for backing to the general public.

A DIFFERENT STRATEGY

Anne Watson and her supporters proceeded very differently in their efforts to establish a birth center in the area. As mentioned previously, Anne was a well-known woman in the community prior to this attempt, with the experience and self-assurance of an active reformer. She was familiar with the local medical scene, including its possibilities and limits for out-of-hospital birthing. She had been director of parent education at a division of the local medical center from 1965 through the mid-1970s. At that time, obstetric services were provided at all three divisions of the medical center, but very few private patients went to the division where she was located. Anne argued that most of the women who came to her division received very poor care. They were routinely given debilitating drugs during labor but were given no information to help them to participate in decision making about their labor and birth experience. While working at this division, Anne acted as a strong consumer advocate and worked to bring about change in routine hospital procedures. She advocated for the decreased use of drugs during labor and delivery, wider dissemination of information to consumers, and the presence of fathers in the delivery room.

During the years that Anne worked at the medical center things changed drastically, largely because of the consolidation of maternity services provided by the medical center. In 1972, all of these services were moved to a new wing at the division where Anne worked. The new facility was very modern and was designed to allow newborns to room with their mothers. Some of the hospital's policies had changed in response to the efforts of Anne and others. At the same time, however, the use of more sophisticated technology and drugs during labor was becoming commonplace.

Anne and her staff in the parent education program were engaged in ongoing conflicts with physicians, labor and delivery nurses, and hospital administrators. Anne's staff, for the most part, did not work in labor and delivery. Rather, they taught in an extensive parent education program that included classes in preparation for childbirth, breastfeeding, and early parenting, among others. The labor and delivery nurses resented the fact that the parent education staff did not have to work shifts in labor and delivery. This resentment, plus a clear disagreement on birthing practices, led to disputes between those nurses who were teaching and those who were working in labor and delivery. There was also a conflict between the parent education staff and the obstetrical department over what constituted appropriate practice in childbirth.

This conflict came to a head when Anne told a local newspaper reporter that one would never find nurse-midwives using forceps during a birth in order to get onto the golf course more quickly. Although the comment was made off the record, it appeared in the local newspaper. According to a chief hospital administrator, whom I will call John Hanson, once it appeared in print there was no question that Anne would be separated from the parent education program and from maternity services in general. Hanson stressed that Anne was not fired from the medical center but was offered a job in pediatrics which she refused. When she left her position, much of her staff in parent education also resigned.

According to John Hanson, Anne Watson had done an outstanding job as director of the parent education program at the medical center for many years. In the two years prior to her resignation, however, the program had been plagued with problems. According to Hanson, these problems were due largely to conflict between the parent education staff and the labor and delivery staff, for which he was willing to blame Anne's people. In his words:

You're talking about a parent support group probably who were on the college campuses in the late '60s, now moving on and perhaps a little older and maybe still full of the zeal that they had on the college campus and trying to channel it in some direction in some positive way and moving from a very happy, very excited new parent into attempting to dictate policy in terms of how things should be done. You've got a lot of things wrapped together in terms of the very active phase of the consumer movement in childbearing circles. And she [Anne Watson] attracted a group of people who—I don't know whether it was deep-seated fear, hatred, jealousy of the medical profession, or not—who began to start dictating or channeling people into the kind of childbearing experience that the experts [the parent education staff] thought they should have.

Hanson expressed great relief that Anne's supporters left along with her:

Thank God that group of instructors left. Thank God they left, because had they stayed on it would have just been dirty, nasty guerrilla warfare for years. But thank God they left, all at once they left. . . . They really did us a favor by resigning, although we honestly did not press them to do that.

A number of the women who resigned from the medical center later became instructors for Childbirth and Parenting Education Associates (CPEA). Childbirth instruction is one of the services which CPEA offers. Many people opt to attend these classes as opposed to those offered through the medical center. According to Hanson, it is those people who go to CPEA's classes who then make unreasonable demands on their doctors.

At the time of the resignations, John Hanson was working behind the scenes with some obstetricians to bring nurse-midwifery training to the medical center. This might have led to practicing privileges for nurse-midwives at the medical center. After the shake-up, however, there was no possibility that that would happen in the foreseeable future.

After leaving the medical center, Anne became director of midwifery services at a birth center in a nearby state. The combination of her experience with opening a birth center and her previous association with the medical center made her well aware of the difficulties which she would face in trying to open a birth center in this area.

Anne understood that the biggest obstacles were finding backup support from a physician and locating a pediatrician who was willing to act as pediatric consultant for the center. Anne entered into formal agreements for such services more than two months before filing her certificate of need application with the state bureau of health planning. By late March 1981, she had an agreement in writing from a well-respected pediatrician to serve as a medical consultant to the center. By early April she had a similar agreement from a popular team of obstetricians with a large and well-respected practice in the area. All of these arrangements were made quietly, without any public discussion or participation. It is possible that Anne knew that she had the support of these physicians at the March meeting with Babyplace, although she made no mention of it at the time.

The original board of directors for the birth center consisted of a president, vice president, secretary, treasurer, and ten members. Of the ten members, five were medical professionals. Anne and her husband agreed to finance personally the purchase of property to house the birth center. The board of directors agreed to lease the property for a five-year period, after which the birth center corporation would have first option to purchase the property. All of these details were taken care of prior to the filing of the certificate of need.

The application was received by the state bureau of health planning in June 1981. After the certificate of need was filed and public announcement was made, there was a customary ten-day period during which anyone could request a public hearing on the matter. Consumers supporting the birth center did not request such a hearing because no opposing groups requested one. Once the ten-day period was over, however, some area physicians asked to be heard by the project review committee. Since the ten-day period had passed, the decision as to whether or not the physicians could be heard was up to the executive director of the health council. He agreed that the physicians could be heard but that Anne Watson would also be asked to attend the hearing.

The hearing for the physicians was held in August 1981. At the hearing a local obstetrician, speaking on behalf of the state obstetrical society and reflecting the views of the American College of Obstetricians and Gynecologists, voiced his strong opposition to the birth center. Among his objections were the following:(1) that the birth center was not, in his opinion, adjacent to an emergency medical facility; (2) that an obstetrician and a pediatrician would not routinely be present at births; (3) that even the backup physicians for the center felt that such services would best be provided within a hospital setting; and (4) that certain medications including intravenous therapy could be used by the nurse-midwives at the center. In a letter to the president of the state medical society, dated September 2, 1981, this same obstetrician detailed his opposition to the birth center. In that letter he concluded:

It appears that a wave of consumer activism has overridden sound medical judgement. I feel it important to write this letter to you so that we have on record our strong feelings on the inadvisability of the birthing project should it come to fruition. The risk to mothers and the newborn is a grave responsibility this group will be inadvisably assuming. Lastly, if indeed this does come to fruition, it would open the door for surgical centers, extension of general health care in small unsupervised facilities in our state once they have set a precedent by their birthing center. The dangers and the problems are obvious.

Also at the August 18 hearing, Anne was attacked by critics who claimed that her motivation for establishing the birth center was revenge against those who had ousted her from her job at the medical center. The usual criticisms that birth centers are unsafe and that nurse-midwives are incompetent caregivers were also raised. Finally, the obstetrician who made the criticisms on behalf of the obstetrical society admitted at the hearing that the primary concern with respect to the birth center was economic. Local obstetricians were concerned with losing business.

On August 25, a subcommittee of the state health council appointed to review the birth center proposal met to discuss the project. This meeting was open to the public, and both physicians and consumers were present. The criticisms made against the birth center by physicians at the August 18 hearing were reiterated. Supporting statements were made on behalf of the birth center by consumers who testified to Anne's competence and compassion. They also spoke about how important they felt the establishment of the birth center was to birthing women, their families, and the community as a whole.

Despite strong opposition from local obstetricians, both the project review committee and the subcommittee approved the birth center. According to the planning assistant who headed the review committee, the medical objections to the project were taken into consideration. The conclusion that was reached at all levels of the approval process, however, was that the birth center would be a good service as well as an alternative to the usual services available in the state. Facilitating the development of alternative obstetrical services was consistent with the goals of the state health plan for 1980–1985 on maternal and child health. The health plan defined alternative services as "any professionally supervised and prepared childbirth experience outside the traditional hospital setting."

The need for alternatives, according to the plan, stemmed from a concern for cost-effective services as well as from an interest in providing services consistent with the needs and desires of the consumer population. The plan states:

> In light of the rapidly rising cost of health care, the scarcity of obstetrical practitioners in certain areas, and recent trends in the delivery of obstetrical services, it is important that the health care system examine all potential methods and arrangements for the delivery of OB [obstetrical] services. Cost effective, quality care that suits the needs of a well-educated consumer population must be assured. This goal seeks to recognize that women have the right to seek care that is not only medically right for themselves and their infants, but that fits their life-styles and respects their individual social, spiritual, and economic needs.

The state health council was made up of a variety of people, including physicians, nurses, health planners and administrators, and academics. Significantly, one of the members of the health council was a vocal supporter of nurse-midwives and birthing centers. She had worked previously with a large urban maternity center and was well aware of the fact that nurse-midwives have a long history of providing excellent care for pregnant and birthing women. The head of the review committee for the birth center actively sought information on birth centers when she could not locate any state or federal guidelines on such facilities. She contacted other birth centers to find out how they operated and what kinds of records they had. She demonstrated her willingness to examine the birth center proposal on its own merits and to approach an unfamiliar concept with an open mind. While she considered the objections raised by physicians, she looked at these objections as representing one position among many.

By September 1981, the approval process for the certificate of need was nearly complete. The physicians, however, continued to record their opposition to the birth center. In a letter to the executive director of the state health council dated September 8, 1981, another local obstetrician stated his opposition to out-of-hospital birth centers. He argued that while there should be free competition in the delivery of health care services, the quality of care should not be diminished. Competition is the best way to insure that services are cost-effective, but a concern for cost-effectiveness should not open the door to "all competitors, licensed or unlicensed, competent or incompetent."

The obvious implication was that the caregivers associated with the birth center were incompetent. The obstetrician concluded by saying that in addition to all the other problems with the birth center proposal, it was also an example of fiscal irresponsibility. On September 16, 1981, a meeting of medical practitioners and social service administrators in the state was held to discuss whether the birth center would be eligible for Medicaid reimbursement. Anne Watson made a presentation to the group explaining her qualifications, the basic organization of a birth center, and the screening process for clients. The physicians were invited to reply to her presentation, and, once again, the obstetrician speaking on behalf of the obstetrical society presented still more objections, including the following: (1) that midwives would not be properly supervised, (2) that childbirth is a very risky undertaking, and (3) that the backup physicians would not have time to oversee the services of the birth center.

In the fall of 1981, Anne Watson received the approval of the state bureau of health planning to proceed with her project but with the stipulation that the birth center have twenty-five thousand dollars in the bank prior to January 1, 1982, the proposed opening date. According to a spokesperson for the health council, the reason for this requirement was to insure the financial stability of the organization and to protect the birth center clientele. While the Health Council required the sum as an indication of the financial stability of the birth center, it agreed ultimately that the entire amount did not have to be in the form of cash but could be partly in the form of other assets.

Following approval of the certificate of need, Anne and her supporters launched a major effort to generate public support for their project. In November 1981, they had a series of three public meetings to inform the community about the center and to appeal for funds needed in order to comply with the health council's financial stipulations.

Each of the meetings followed the same format. Anne explained that the birth center represented the first attempt to bring this out-of-hospital birthing option to the state. At the birth center, the emphasis would be on birth as a healthy process requiring little or no intervention. The birthing woman would be in control. Anne stressed the fact that the costs for maternity care would be much lower at the birth center than they were at the local hospital.

According to Anne, the birth center is meant to be an adaptation of the home environment for low-risk women who wish to have a natural birth. No medication is given routinely during labor, no forceps are used, and of course, no Cesarean births occur at the center. Mothers and babies usually remain there from four to twelve hours after birth.

Anne explained that all births at the center would be attended by nurse-midwives, professionally trained nurses who have additional training in midwifery and certification from the American College of Nurse-Midwives; she added that nurse-midwives are "experts in normal maternity care." If an abnormal situation arises, either during pregnancy or during labor, clients are transferred to the care of the physicians who provide backup support for the center.

In order to be eligible for a birth center birth, a woman must be in good health and must have no history of obstetrical problems. Women between the ages of fifteen and thirty-five are eligible for care for a first baby. Women up to forty years of age are eligible for subsequent births. The nurse-midwife argued that the vast majority of women are candidates for birth centers. About 85 percent of women are able to give birth in the out-of-hospital setting.

Anne stressed the fact that once a woman is admitted to the center in labor, there would be a nurse-midwife with her throughout her labor and birth. If another woman is admitted to the center at the same time, a second nurse-midwife would be called. There is a strong belief among nurse-mid-wives about the importance of this one-to-one contact between the nurse-midwife and the birthing woman. This differs markedly from standard treatment by a physician in a hospital. A physician may not be present at all during the early stages of labor when care is provided largely or exclusively by labor and delivery nurses. The same physician might be attending several women at once.

Following the brief overview on nurse-midwives and birth centers, a film on contemporary midwifery practices entitled *Daughters of Time* was shown. The film was followed by a panel discussion with parents who had had babies at a birth center in an adjacent state, the closest such facility. While all of the couples were from the local area, they had all chosen to travel about one hour for all prenatal care as well as for labor and birth in order to have a birth center experience. All of the parents described the comfortable homelike atmosphere and the strong support of the nurse-midwives. One of the couples had previously had a hospital birth but opted for a birth center the second time because they did not want to repeat their hospital experience. They said that the hospital birth had been a totally dehumanizing experience over which they had no control. The birth center birth was very different. They could have their first child present for the birth as well as other family and friends. They were able to choose the circumstances surrounding the birth and were glad for the opportunity for closeness with their newborn immediately following birth.

After brief presentations from all of the panelists, questions were taken from the audience. Attendance at each of the three meetings ranged from about twenty to forty people, some of whom were already birth center supporters. Most of the questions from the audience had to do with how competent and confident panel members felt about having a birth outside of the hospital and about judging the condition of a newborn so shortly after birth. The panel members explained that they were well prepared for childbirth and that they were taught infant assessment techniques since they would be taking their newborns home within twelve hours following birth.

Those who attended seemed sincerely interested in gaining more information about birth centers but generally did not seem totally convinced about the wisdom of out-of-hospital births. While there was an audience for all of the public meetings, it was small at each of them. It was clear that there was some public interest and support, but also that the supporters of the birth center would have to convince more people of the superiority of this alternative to hospital births if they were going to be able to generate the clientele needed for the center to survive.

At the time of the public meetings in November, the center already had its first client, who was due to give birth in March 1982. The issue of third-party reimbursement was still unresolved and continued to be so throughout the center's first year of operation. Once the certificate of need had been approved, however, reimbursement from Blue Cross became likely. Initially, Blue Cross had said that it would require a physician to be present for each birth, which was contrary to the intended operation of the birth center. Subsequently, the Blue Cross regulation was changed to reflect state law, which required that nurse-midwives have a written alliance with a physician who would supply backup support; it was understood, however, that a physician would not be present for births which occurred at the center. During the center's first year of operation, approval for Blue Cross reimbursement occurred on a case-by-case basis. In the meantime, Blue Cross/Blue Shield worked on offering birth center services as a rider to its existing contracts with local employers. If an employer wanted to make the birth center option available to its employees, for example, it would have to request that particular rider to the standard contract. The rider was going to be made free upon request because the fees for birth center services were about half of those for a hospital birth, and the center would therefore be cost-effective for Blue Cross/Blue Shield.

In February 1982, the birth center opened its doors. The weeks before the opening were a flurry of volunteer activity. The ardent group of supporters who had helped to see this project through were involved in a variety of activities to prepare for opening day. People painted, sewed curtains, and hung potted plants; they also donated furniture and various household items, including dishes and pots and pans. While there was no guarantee at this point of how long the center would remain open, Anne and her supporters had been successful in reaching their goal: establishing a birth center in the area.

DISCUSSION

The single most crucial factor which contributed to the successful opening of the birth center was Anne's ability to generate support from a team of physicians. Without it the project would have been stymied. Because this support came from one of the largest, most popular, and well-respected obstetrical practices in the area, it was very hard for those physicians in opposition to make a strong case against the center. They certainly tried to block the opening, but they were limited with regard to the tactics that they could use. They could not attack the backup physicians as unfit or incompetent or threaten them with the loss of hospital privileges. The opposition was left, then, with secondary criticisms, such as that the backup physicians would be too busy to oversee this service or that the service would be too far from the medical center. Opponents were in no position to force the center's backup support to withdraw from the project, which would have been necessary in order to stop the center from opening.

There were two primary reasons why Anne was able to gain support from the physicians while Babyplace was not. The first had to do with her status as a certified health professional. While the members of Babyplace were all consumers with no medical training or credentials, Anne was a trained, licensed health care practitioner seeking a contractual alliance with a physician in accordance with the provisions of state law. There was little, if any, possibility of a physician agreeing to enter into an alliance with consumers. While the philosophy which has guided the birth center is certainly at odds with the dominant childbirth practices which routinely use sophisticated technology to monitor labors, it does not fall completely outside of the medical model. Anne Watson frequently refers to herself as an "expert in normal maternity care." While she clearly respects her clients and their rights to participate in shaping their own birth experiences, she does not reject the notion of expertise. Rather, she views expertise in birthing care as a kind of continuum ranging from the ability to handle normal births to the ability to handle pathological cases. Certain routine problems fall within the realm of her expertise. Other conditions and problems (twin births, forceps deliveries, Cesarean sections) require the expertise of physicians with more training and experience with birth pathology. Although Anne is critical of the medical model of birth, she herself is a licensed medical professional. Her professional status gave her a certain amount of credibility within the medical community.

Second, Anne was able to gain physician support as a result of her personal history at the medical center. She had known the head of her backup team for a number of years while she worked there. While she was always the subject of some controversy, she also had the reputation of doing an excellent job as coordinator of a large parent education program, of being a strong consumer advocate, and of fighting for more progressive policies at the medical center. The team of doctors who agreed to support the birth center also have a reputation as consumer advocates and have been labeled by some as being too willing to cater to the wishes of their patients. As one hospital administrator put it, they "have always been regarded by some of their colleagues as being more supportive of the whimsical demands of their patients than others are willing to be." While it would probably be hard to get anyone to admit it, there were probably some obstetricians who were glad this team of doctors would be available to deal with the "kooks" and "raving lunatics."

Anne's history at the medical center was, of course, a double-edged sword. It enabled her to make the connections necessary for her to open the birth center. However, she also had made a number of enemies during her tenure and had a reputation as a troublemaker among certain segments of the obstetrical community. Fear of opposition grounded in hostilities toward her often led her to work very quietly behind the scenes with a small group of supporters, making no public announcement about her activities until her success was assured. This can sometimes be an effective strategy. At other times, however, it can be a very serious mistake. This dilemma will be discussed later with respect to a malpractice insurance crisis which the birth center found itself facing three years after it opened.

Another important factor which contributed to the success of the birth center was the positive reaction of the state health council. The person in charge of the project for the council was interested in the birth center concept and impressed with Anne Watson. The certificate of need application was skillfully prepared and contained documentation which demonstrated that the project could succeed if the certificate of need were approved. Most important, however, was the fact that the birth center alternative was cost-effective and consistent with the goals of the health council. At the time of the center's opening, the cost for maternity care (prenatal care, labor and delivery services, and postnatal care including a home visit) was nine hundred dollars—about one-half the cost of a routine hospital birth. While the center's fees have continued to rise over its years of operation, they remain roughly half of the standard hospital fees. The following quote from the state's health plan reflects the strong interest in cost-effective services:

In [this state], obstetrical services are provided under the direction of physicians and, with rare exceptions, deliveries take place in a hospital setting. No alternative care is available. There is considerable evidence from other states that the low risk population can receive adequate, safe care through the utilization of more cost-effective, less technologically sophisticated alternatives. As physicians and other health care providers become more aware of the need for family-centered alternatives, the need for qualified midwives, birthing rooms, and birth centers to deliver such care should increase.

The fact that birth centers are cost-effective seems to be as significant as anything else about them. This is not to imply that the health council was willing to sacrifice quality care for lower costs, but rather to suggest that cost containment was and continues to be an important consideration among health planners. Their reaction to the birth center and alternative birth arrangements generally might have been very different if their costs were more in line with standard hospital costs.

As stated earlier, the state health plan explicitly limits its definition of alternative childbirth services to those which are professionally supervised by licensed practitioners. While the plan certainly reflects a desire to promote services which meet a range of consumer interests and lifestyles, it makes it very clear that these services should be provided by professional medical personnel. The proposal for a birth center which was presented by Anne combined the health council's goals of meeting consumer demands and at the same time promoting professionally supervised services. Again, the fact that those involved with Babyplace were consumers worked against them.

In addition to not having medical credentials, the Babyplace group also lacked the necessary background and experience with the day-to-day operation of a birth center which would have been helpful in putting together the certificate of need. Babyplace also did not have access to the financial resources needed to start a center and to satisfy the health council.

Birth centers are not typically lucrative ventures, but Anne and her group had considerably more financial resources at their disposal than did Babyplace. Anne and her spouse were in a position to finance personally the property which would house the center. Much of the initial renovation was done by volunteers (as was much of the work involved in running the center). Money still needed to be raised, however, and although finding the initial funds was somewhat difficult, birth center supporters were able to put together enough money to open their facility.

The members of Babyplace were particularly inept politically. The professional support that they needed would have been difficult for any consumer group to attain. But Babyplace made political mistakes at every turn, including alienating groups such as CPEA and nursing mothers organizations which were likely sources of support.

Anne and her supporters, on the other hand, clearly understood the politics surrounding their efforts to open a birth center. They realized that they would face strong opposition from the obstetrical community. For this reason, they proceeded quietly and cautiously until they were able to secure written support from a pediatrician and a team of obstetricians. Given her history at the medical center, Anne knew the most likely sources of opposition to her efforts. She also knew that opposition to the birth center had little to do with concern with maintaining the quality of maternity care and everything to do with maintaining the authority and control of physicians and hospitals over childbirth.

This interest was reflected in the letters and statements by physicians in response to the certificate of need application. There was great concern that a physician would not be present for every birth and that nonphysicians would be in a position to determine birthing protocol in an out-of-hospital setting, to administer drugs, and to completely oversee the care of birthing women. The implication was strong that nurse-midwives were incompetent practitioners and that permitting them to open a facility such as a birth center flew in the face of sound medical judgment. Furthermore, opposing physicians claimed that if nurse-midwives were allowed to open a birth center, this would pave the way for a host of pseudomedical personnel to set up unsupervised facilities throughout the state.

Similar attitudes were expressed by the medical center administrator John Hanson. He insisted that the medical center had no set policy regarding how women should give birth and that it would have been inappropriate for the hospital to dictate what kind of childbirth experience people should have. His comments, however, reflect an underlying contempt toward childbirth activists and toward women in general:

> What I mean is all the heat and all the activists in the community, all the people who are willing to say to you, you must have a natural childbirth, you should not have an episiotomy, you should never take medication, and on and on and on, are the very people who will say the hospital is doing those ugly things to you. Hell, it doesn't make any difference to us . . . it's your baby! You've hired a guy to help you have that baby and you ought to ask him the questions and if you don't like the answers you ought to find yourself another doctor. You can deliver on a grass mat standing on your head for all we care.

In studying the formation of this birth center, it becomes clear that there was some convergence between the medical model and the birth center project. It was founded in an environment largely dominated by medical experts, laws which favored the medical model, insurance constraints, and cultural beliefs rooted in technocratic ideology. The birth center incorporates some aspects of the medical model, including a belief in the importance of medical professionalism and in a professional hierarchy based on expert knowledge as well as a belief in the use of cost-effectiveness as a criterion for health care decision making. These shared beliefs provided the basis for approval of the birth center project by the health council.

At the same time, there is also significant divergence between the medical model and the birth center. The philosophy of birth which guides practice at the birth center is rooted in the midwifery model, which sees birth as a healthy process and as a woman-centered activity. Anne says that when she looks at a pregnant woman, she sees a healthy woman experiencing a healthy life process. This view differs sharply from the medical definition of birth as pathology.

Clearly there are some ambiguities and conflicts to consider in this case. On the one hand, Anne Watson was successful in establishing a birth center despite some vocal protests from the medical community. On the other hand, the context in which the birth center has been established is one in which the power and authority of physicians and hospitals is maintained. The birth center cannot function without physician backup. The local medical center denies practicing privileges to certified nurse-midwives, so continuity of care for hospital transfers is limited. Nurse-midwives can stay with women who are transferred from the birth center, but they cannot act as birth attendants.

Questions emerge about power, authority, and control. In what ways does the establishment of the birth center affect the power of birthing women to control their birthing experiences? In what ways does the existence of the birth center affect the power of the medical establishment? These are discussed in the following chapters.

7

The Operation
of the Birth Center

INTRODUCTION

In discussing the formation of the birth center, I showed that the center shares some basic organizational and ideological features with the medical model. The birth center is attached to mainstream medicine through the backup physician and through Anne's professional training and status. While she often finds herself in direct opposition to the medical establishment, her status as a certified nurse-midwife distinguishes her from lay midwives in the state and enhances her credibility. Beyond these features, legal and insurance constraints force the birth center to accommodate to some degree to the dominant model. In this way, the center exists within a set of elite-controlled institutions. At the same time, practice at the birth center, the patterns of interpersonal relations, and the quality of childbirth are woman-centered, relatively egalitarian, and focused on enhancing the birth experience for women and families. The birth center provides an environment for childbirth which is qualitatively different from the hospital and which has met with extremely positive responses from birth center clients. The existence of the birth center not only broadens the range of alternatives available for child-bearing women but also opens up the possibility for more radical alternatives. Yet it is also true that just as some conformity to the medical model was necessary for the formation of the birth center, that model continues to impose constraints upon the operation of the center.

This chapter portrays the actual day-to-day life of the birth center. It talks about its clients and their experiences, and includes testimony from some of the women who have given birth at the center.

The birth center opened its doors in February 1982. As pointed out in the previous chapter, volunteers pitched in to prepare the center for opening. Many of the women and men who had supported Anne in her efforts to open the birth center participated in a variety of tasks. People painted, scrubbed, sewed, and decorated day and night to get things ready. There was a great sense of celebration and anticipation among the volunteers. People felt a real sense of accomplishment for having succeeded in getting the support needed to open the center and for having transformed an old three-story residence into a warm, comfortable place for women and their families. There were 77 births during the first year. Of the first 100 births, 13 were transferred to the medical center. Of the hospital transfers, one was a breech delivery, six were prolonged labors, and six were Cesarean sections. During the second year there were 115 births, and by the third year the number of births increased to 155. The most births within a one-year period occurred in 1990, when there were 187 births. The number of births has dropped more recently. In 1993 there were 133 births and in 1994 there were 139.

BASIC OPERATION OF THE BIRTH CENTER

In the summer of 1982, I worked at the birth center as a receptionist and general all-around helper in order to observe the operation of the center and the interactions between midwives and clients and to gain information about the clientele.

I would usually begin my day by pulling the files for the clients who would be seen that day. The primary activity on most days was seeing clients for prenatal visits and for well-woman checkups. I would greet people when they came in and make appointments as they were leaving. I also took phone calls from prospective clients and scheduled them for orientation sessions, and took calls from expectant and new mothers who had questions for Anne and her partner. In addition, I would sometimes do laundry, sterilize instruments, and help out with anything around the center which needed doing.

At the time, the staff of the birth center consisted of Anne Watson, a second nurse-midwife whom I will call Becky, a registered nurse, and another volunteer who did typing and general office work. Anne served as medical director of the center, provided prenatal care and well-woman checkups, and attended births. When the birth center opened Anne was in her early fifties. She had worked as a nurse and a certified nurse-midwife for more than twenty years. She had served as head of the parent education program at the local medical center and she was also the founder of the first chapter of a nursing mothers group in the state. She had long been recognized as an advocate for pregnant and birthing women. She was well known among nurse-midwives in the region and highly respected by her supporters, her backup physicians, and her pediatric physician. Becky joined the birth center a few months after it opened. In her early thirties, she had recently married and had moved from a southern state where she had been involved in another birth center. The registered nurse, whom I will call Emma, was a local woman in her late twenties who was the mother of two young children and was pregnant with her third child. I asked her if she was planning on having her baby at the birth center, and she hesitated a moment before telling me that she was planning a home birth. It was through Emma that I was able to make contact with one of the lay midwives attending home births in the state. The other volunteer was a woman who had had her second baby at Anne's first birth center. She had been a strong supporter of Anne's efforts to open a center and continued to show her support by volunteering.

While Anne Watson is still the director of the birth center, staff members have changed over the years. There have been a number of midwives and nurses who have worked at the center. At the beginning office work was done by volunteers. Eventually, however, a staff person was hired to do this work. The nurse-midwives at the center are supported by a team of physicians who provide consultation and backup as well as by a pediatric consultant.

The birth center is a detached three-story residential building in the middle of a residential city street. Most of the other houses on the street are attached or semi-detached houses. When the center first opened, it was a relatively small space with only one birthing room in operation. The second floor of the birth center was not yet renovated. In 1985 a three-story addition was added to the back of the center, resulting in the large functional building which now houses the center.

On the first floor of the center there is a waiting room, a small office area, two examining rooms, the director's office, a small kitchen, a powder room, and one birth room with an adjoining bathroom. The second floor has two birth rooms and a bathroom, a small TV room, a large kitchen/dining room, and a family room. The third floor has a large all-purpose room with a kitchen area which is used for meetings, classes, and social gatherings. It also has a bedroom and bath that are sometimes used by student nurse-midwives who do their practicums at the birth center.

The rooms are decorated in a comfortable, homelike fashion. Over the years clients and supporters have donated a variety of things which contribute to the center's warmth. One family donated an antique oak bed which is used in one of the birth rooms. Another family contributed a rocking chair to commemorate a lost pregnancy and to stand as a symbol of thanks for the care Anne provided through this difficult time and of hope for future

children. Other clients have done stenciling, needlepoint, and art work for
the various birth rooms.

When prospective clients express an interest in or seek information about
the birth center, they are scheduled for an orientation session given by one
of the nurse-midwives. At the orientation a nurse-midwife explains that the
birth center is a short-stay maternity care facility with a homelike atmosphere.
While there is access to hospital care through the backup physicians should
this become necessary, births at the center are unmedicated and allowed to
progress without interference. Electronic fetal heart monitors are not used to
monitor heart rates, labors are not induced or augmented, forceps are not
used, and of course, Cesarean sections are not performed. While invasive
technologies and drugs are not used, labors are monitored very closely by the
nurse-midwives. A nurse-midwife remains with each woman throughout her
labor. Maternal and fetal heart rates are checked often, as is the progress of
the labor. Mothers are encouraged to drink lots of liquids (juices, water, ice
chips, fruit popsicles) during labor and are reminded to follow the procedures
stressed in childbirth classes of changing position frequently, urinating at least
once per hour, and relaxing as much as possible. All birth center clients are
required to attend childbirth classes. These classes are offered at the center
itself and included in the basic fee.

About 85 percent of those women who register at the center go on to give
birth there. About 8 percent are transferred to a physician's care due to
complications which arise during pregnancy. Another 7 percent are transferred to the hospital during labor. About 3 to 4 percent of birth center clients
have Cesarean sections. When women are transferred to the hospital during
labor, their attending nurse-midwife goes and stays with them during labor
and birth. Nurse-midwives do not have practicing privileges at the local
medical center, but they do provide care and support to birth center clients
when a transfer occurs.

At the orientation session it is explained that birthing women are encouraged to participate actively in their own care and in choosing the circumstances for their birthing experiences. They may invite anyone they like,
including other children, to be present at the birth. Clients are encouraged
to mark the event in the way that seems most appropriate for them. Many
want to record the birth through photographs and/or videotape. The center
has video cameras available for use by clients for a small rental fee. Many
families celebrate after the birth with a special meal which they have prepared
and brought with them to the center. Clients are free to do whatever feels
comfortable and right for them. Women are free to choose their own position
for giving birth. There is a Jacuzzi available to use for relaxation during labor.
Clients may choose to play music which they enjoy or find relaxing. Birthing

women and their families have control over what they want their birthing experience to be like.

Once the basic philosophy and operation of the center are explained, a tour of the center is conducted and prospective clients are encouraged to ask questions. The nurse-midwives stress that the reason for the orientation is to acquaint people with the birth center and allow them to decide for themselves whether they feel comfortable with this approach. After a woman has attended an orientation session she can schedule an initial visit. About 90 percent of those who attend an orientation session do become birth center clients.

During the initial visit, a nurse-midwife takes a thorough medical history of the pregnant woman as well as any pertinent information on other family members. A nurse-midwife conducts a thorough physical examination complete with standard lab and blood tests such as a Pap smear and hematocrit. As on every subsequent visit, the midwife will listen for the fetal heartbeat, usually with a doptone, a device which amplifies the heartbeat and allows anyone present to hear it. My desk was located along the wall dividing the examination room from the reception area, and the amplification was often enough for me to hear the heartbeat along with the delighted squeals and joyous cries of prospective parents. It is important to note that fathers (or any other support persons the mother wishes) are strongly encouraged to participate in the pregnancy and to attend any or all prenatal visits. Many fathers do participate throughout the pregnancy and find this to be extremely important and rewarding.

Based upon the information gathered at the initial visit, the midwife decides whether a woman is an appropriate client for the birth center. As long as a woman does not have any of the characteristics that would place her in a high-risk category, and the vast majority of women do not, she is accepted as a client. It is important to note, however, that the nurse-midwives use the same criteria for determining the high-risk patient as an obstetrician would use. Among the conditions or characteristics which would define a woman as high risk are chronic disease (heart disease or neurological, renal, endocrine, hypertensive, or metabolic disorders), diabetes, and multiple pregnancy.

At about the twentieth week of pregnancy, each first-time birth center client is seen by one of the center's backup physicians. The physician examines the woman to determine whether she is an appropriate candidate for a birth center delivery. I am not aware of a single case in which the backup physician contradicted the judgment of the nurse-midwife.

At the first visit, the pregnant woman is instructed on how to conduct her own urinalysis to check for the presence of protein and/or sugar in the urine. After this initial instruction, she is expected to repeat this test on each subsequent visit and report the results to the nurse-midwife. The client is also expected to check her weight at each visit and report it to the midwife, who records it on the weight chart. Nurse-midwives are careful to remind clients that they are free to look through their files at any time. The files belong to the clients. There is nothing secret in them, and clients should not hesitate to look through them whenever they wish. Clients are also informed that one of the most important parts of each prenatal visit is asking questions, talking about doubts or confusion, and clarifying points of information. The initial visit takes about one hour, and subsequent visits usually about a half hour. Visits are never rushed and clients are rarely kept waiting more than a few minutes before an appointment.

The single most important aspect of prenatal care as far as the nurse-midwives are concerned is nutrition. Women are encouraged to follow a high-protein diet of about 2,200 calories per day. Each client is given a diet to follow which contains information on necessary intake of fruits, vegetables, fats, carbohydrates, and protein. Women who are pregnant for the first time are requested to record everything they eat for two twenty-four hour periods. This record is then reviewed with the nurse-midwife to see if nutritional intake is adequate. Any problems or difficulties are discussed.

According to the medical model, prenatal care is something which a pregnant woman gets from a physician or other caregiver during a number of visits throughout her pregnancy. According to the nurse-midwives at the birth center, however, prenatal care is something that pregnant women give themselves twenty-four hours a day throughout a pregnancy. Clients at the birth center are therefore supplied with a great deal of information to help them insure a healthy pregnancy and a healthy baby. For instance, all clients are provided with a booklet that gives dietary information, including nutritional requirements for pregnant women and lists of good sources of protein and iron. There is also a section on common complaints of pregnancy, causes, and recommended remedies. For nausea and vomiting, for example, the booklet recommends small, frequent meals, soda crackers, and an increase in vitamin B-6. Clients are also told about circumstances when particular symptoms warrant a call to one of the nurse-midwives. Some leg swelling, for example, can be a common occurrence during pregnancy, but if swelling is excessive clients should call the center, especially if it is accompanied by swelling in the hands and/or the face. The booklet also offers information on exercises during pregnancy, the benefits of relaxation, and some facts on smoking and pregnancy. The end of the booklet contains information on labor, birth, and newborn care. Information, then, is not used as a source of power against the client. Rather, it is viewed as something to be shared in order to enhance the childbearing experience of each individual woman.

Throughout the birth center's years of operation, the educational component of its services has increased. Initially most of the information was supplied at the prenatal visits and at classes on preparation for childbirth. These classes, however, were not taught at the center itself. Rather, birth center clients went to classes offered by Childbirth and Parenting Education Associates (CPEA). Childbirth classes are now offered by the center. In some respects this represents an improvement over the initial arrangement, because all of those in the birth center class are preparing for a birth center experience and the classes can be geared accordingly. It is also important because childbirth classes are now used to strengthen and reinforce relations among women at the center. Taught by one of the nurses at the center, the classes provide an opportunity for clients to build a relationship with the nurse teaching the class as well as with each other. However, because birth center clients do not attend classes open to the public, the visibility of the birth center in the community at large is decreased.

The center now offers, in addition, an early pregnancy series consisting of classes in (1) fetal development, (2) nutrition, (3) common and uncommon developments during pregnancy, and (4) exercise and relaxation. There is also a class on assessing maternal and infant health in the days immediately following birth. All of these classes are included in the basic birth center fee.

For those families who wish to have other children attend the birth, the center offers a sibling preparation class. At the class, children are given some idea about what to expect at a birth—some of the sounds they might hear and some of the things they might see, such as fluid and blood. The class instructors fill a balloon with water to serve as a model for the amniotic sac. They then pop the "sac" with a pin to show how the "fluid" runs out once the sac breaks. This is a particularly popular part of the class. Children are shown all of the instruments which might be used at a birth and are encouraged to look at them and touch them if they wish. Questions and discussion are also encouraged. Children who do attend birth have a support person—a grandparent, an aunt or an uncle, or a family friend—who cares for the child throughout the labor and birth. Children may be in the room throughout the labor and birth if they are comfortable and if their mother is comfortable with this. Anytime that children wish to leave the room and go to another part of the center, they are free to do so and their support persons are available to care for them. The center is large and child friendly, with plenty of room for playing, watching TV or videos, eating a meal, or taking a nap.

When my daughter was born at the birth center, my husband and I planned to have our son, then four years old, attend the birth. He enjoyed the preparation class very much and was eager to discuss all he knew about birth with the instructors. As things turned out, my labor progressed very quickly, and my daughter was born only ten minutes after I arrived at the center. My parents were on their way to the center with my son, but they did not arrive until shortly after the birth. Although my son was not present for the birth, he did meet his sister within a half hour of her birth. He held her and brought her a stuffed animal. He laid next to her on the bed while she was examined by the nurse. After the exam, my husband and I and our children all snuggled together in the big oak bed where my daughter was born. Our son felt very much a part of his sister's birth, just as we had planned for and anticipated together. It was a wonderful experience for all of us to have him so involved.

Other birth center parents expressed similar views about having siblings present at birth:

> Preparation included accompanying us to prenatal visits, where he was very accepted. He helped measure Mom's tummy, feel the baby, and hold the amplifier when listening to the fetal heartbeat. He called it the "heart beeps." The people and surroundings became very comfortable and familiar. . . . Jason helped pack a suitcase for the new baby, planned a sibling gift exchange, and planned activities to do with his sponsor, like bake chocolate chip cookies during labor, which was very special to him, [and] passing them all around after the birth.

Another mother described this experience:

> I began pushing at 11:45 P.M. and it was extremely painful. Despite Sam's preparation for the birth I still had some reservations about his watching. As long as I was in control I had no problem, but when I started pushing I wasn't so sure. . . . After a couple of pushes I felt more confident and sent for Sam. He came racing down the hall with Susan [his support person] as soon as he heard the baby was coming. Perched on a stool at the foot of the bed, being tightly held by his Aunt Susan, Sam watched and waited. I prayed Sam was all right and I wanted so to see the expression on his face. But in my deep concentration I was unable to open my eyes. My only reassurance that he was okay was hearing Susan's attentive voice. She gently assured him over and over, saying, "Mommy's okay, she's working real hard. See the baby's head? The baby is going to come soon!" Repeating this to Sam over and over again, she spoke constantly, not giving him a chance to worry or think negatively.

Not all birth center clients want their other children present for birth. Some prefer to have children come shortly after birth to meet their new sibling.

Most clients who have other children do include them in some significant way in the events surrounding birth.

The philosophy of birth which guides practice at the birth center is woman-centered. The well-being of the pregnant woman is viewed as central for her own sake as well as to insure the health of her child. Furthermore, women are strongly encouraged to determine the circumstances of their births and to actively participate in their own care. The philosophy of the nurse-midwives encourages birthing women and their partners to be active partici-pants in shaping their birth experiences.

The relationships which I observed between the nurse-midwives and clients were friendly and devoid of the formality which often characterizes the physi-cian-patient relationship. Everyone was on a first name basis, and the atmos-phere was warm, supportive, and relaxed. Upon arriving for my first day of work, for example, I found Anne having coffee with a new mother, father, and grandmother. As they sipped coffee, the nurse-midwife went over some infor-mation on checking the baby after the family returned home. It was 9:00 A.M. and the baby had been born seven hours earlier at 2:00 A.M., but Anne was still with this new family. After they all finished their coffee, the new mother took a shower and the family headed for home.

During my observations, I witnessed countless examples of this kind of support being provided by the nurse-midwives. One morning a woman called about a problem with a fussy baby. Anne Watson spoke to this woman in an extremely reassuring and sympathetic way, as someone who had herself experienced the doubts and worries that the woman was expressing. Anne told the woman to nap when the baby napped and to forget about the housework. She told the mother that when her husband got home from work to have him take the baby so that she could have a short time to relax. Anne took her time with this woman and asked how things were going otherwise. Listening to the conversation, one would have thought that she had no other demands on her time. I knew, however, that she was in the middle of an extremely busy morning. She conveyed a genuine interest in the woman's problem, and their conversation was not characterized by distance or formality.

BIRTH CENTER CLIENTELE

While working at the center I collected some basic data on a sample of thirty-four clients and their partners. This data was collected from clients when they registered at the center. Of the thirty-four couples, nineteen had previous children, while fifteen were expecting first births. The clients ranged in age from 19 to 33, with the majority falling between the ages of 24 and

28. Three had had a previous birth at a birth center or at home. Only one of the couples in the sample was black; the rest were white. While eight of the couples were uninsured, twenty-six had health insurance that covered birth center services.

Those in the sample gave a number of different reasons for coming to the center, but the most common reason, mentioned by ten of the women, was a dislike for hospitals or a previous bad experience with a hospital birth. Five women said that they wanted a birth center experience. Of the three who had a previous birth center or home birth experience, all listed that experience as their reason for seeking a birth center the second time around. The one woman who had had a home birth said that she felt the birth center was a better alternative.

There were a number of other responses listed as reasons for coming to the center, including a desire to have siblings present at birth, a preference for a "natural birth," a desire to have a nurse-midwife as a birth attendant, and the lack of health insurance. Since the birth center fees are about half of those for a hospital birth, this might be a particularly attractive choice for those who are not covered by insurance. Of the eight in the sample who had no insurance coverage, however, only two listed this as their reason for coming to the birth center.

Most of those in the sample said that they were referred to the center by a friend, but other referrals came from the backup physicians, the local chapter of Planned Parenthood, the state health council, Childbirth and Parenting Education Associates, and the local newspaper.

Of those who gave information on their educational background, seven were high school graduates, five had some college, seven were college graduates, and two had some graduate education. There was a similar spread with regard to occupations, which ranged from waitress to engineer and included day care provider, registered nurse, social worker, home-maker, designer, salesperson, and carpenter. This sample of birth center clients is almost exclusively white. They range from working class to upper middle class. Within this group there were no particular characteristics which might be used to explain why these people opted for this type of birthing experience.

Nelson (1986) argues that in her comparisons of the desires of middle-class and working-class women regarding childbirth, middle-class women wanted births free from medical intervention in which they could be fully involved. Working-class women wanted a more passive role and more medical inter-vention. Nelson uses education as the defining characteristic of class. Those with no more than a high school diploma were categorized as working class. Those with at least four years of college were categorized as middle class.

Those who fell somewhere in between were categorized on the basis of the job they held.

This method of defining class is questionable. But if I apply Nelson's categories to my own sample, there is an equal split between those with high school diplomas and those with college degrees. Beyond this, a number of people held jobs that could be classified as working class. All birth center clients are conscious of the type of birth experience that they want and, even more particularly, of the type of experience they are rejecting. This is not a choice which is limited only to those who are highly educated or solidly middle class, although it is the case that clients at the center which I studied do tend to be more highly educated than the general population.

The data from the National Birth Center Study compiled by Rooks et al. (1989) does demonstrate that birth center clients generally tend to be more highly educated than the larger population of women giving birth. Among the birth center population, for example, 31.8 percent of the women had sixteen or more years of education, compared with 18.7 percent of the general population of birthing women. It is worth noting, however, that 32.3 percent of women in the birth center sample had twelve years of education and 12.4 percent had less than that.

It was mentioned above that thirty-three of the couples in the sample were white, while only one was black. There were no Hispanic or Asian couples in this sample, which accurately reflects the fact that the birth center clientele is overwhelmingly white. While the staff of the birth center has changed somewhat over its five-year history, all of the members have been white. The same is true for the board of directors, medical consultants, and everyone else in a decision-making role for the center. While the clientele of the birth center has been large enough to keep it going for the past several years, the center has never operated to capacity and is always seeking new clients. Despite the fact that the neighborhood surrounding the center has a largely black and Hispanic population, no specific effort has ever been made to attract these people to the center. Over the years that the center has been open, I have never heard any discussion about targeting the population around the center as a source of additional business, despite a great concern about the fact that the number of births per year at the center has now leveled off.

The fact that so few birth center clients are black in a city with a large black population begs explanation. It appears that a message is being sent to the black community that they are not welcome at the center. While it does not seem that this is intentional on the part of the birth center staff, the fact that all of the center's decision makers and most of the clientele are white creates a distinct impression that blacks are excluded. In the course of my research, I have heard many childbirth activists criticize the birth center movement for being race- and class-biased. While the class background of clients at this birth center represents a range from working-class to upper-class, there are few clients who could be classified as poor, and there is almost no racial diversity among the client population.

While the data in this sample is limited in scope, it reflects the findings presented by Rooks et al. (1989) regarding race and education of birth center clientele. This data challenges the argument that only the highly educated consumer will question dominant birth practices and seek out alternatives.

BIRTH STORIES

Those who do come to the birth center for prenatal care, labor, and birth report very positive experiences. The following birth stories from the center's newsletter offer examples of the experiences which birthing women and their families have there.

Nancy's Story

Labor began differently than it did with my firstborn, Fabio. With him, contractions hit like bad cramps, not too severe, but enough that I knew I was in labor. They advanced quickly and within three hours I was at the hospital with three-minute contractions. I laid in bed waiting for my husband, Lawrence, to come, and remember giggling because I was tickled at how well I was keeping in control, even amidst the screams from some of the other laboring women.

Lawrence arrived just before transition and applied all the little tricks learned in class. He was so helpful, massaging me, applying cool, wet cloths to my face, giving me licks from a lollipop to help ease my dry mouth, and, most importantly, reminding me to slow down my breathing. At about four hours into my labor it was time to push, which I was not at all good at, but my nurse got me straightened out. She reminded me of a football coach, shouting out play by play. I don't think I would have done half as well without her.

I remember thinking what a bother it was to labor in one room, hop onto the stretcher to push, and then scoot onto the delivery table. Legs in stirrups, sterile sheets in place, a cold disinfectant being splashed on my bottom—all this while I was trying so hard to push the baby down. How I wished a birthing room was available! The doctor scrubbed up, took an instrument, and ruptured my membranes. After an episiotomy, one good push and out came the baby's head. Another good push and the rest of our son flowed out.

It felt so warm and I couldn't believe that the pain was over. A total of five and a half hours of labor and delivery—not bad for my first time.

Now with my second baby, Sophia, I wasn't so sure what was going on. She was due August 4, and on August 3, our seventh wedding anniversary, contractions began at 9:15 A.M. while on our way to breakfast. I assumed it was a contraction since it was stronger than a Braxton-Hicks, though not at all painful. I didn't tell Lawrence until the second came fifteen minutes later, but I said to remain calm and not to hurry through breakfast because they weren't strong. They went on all day. The contractions weren't painful, but a real nuisance.

I spoke with Mary [the midwife] at 7:00 P.M. and she said to rest and that it just wasn't time. We decided to visit my mother and as soon as we walked through her door at 8:00 P.M. the first strong contraction hit. They continued every ten minutes and we left to go home at 9:10 P.M. At home, contractions were six minutes apart and severe, and I was really using my breathing techniques. I called Mary, said we were on our way, called Fabio's support person, his aunt JoAnne, and we were off. We went by JoAnne's, she followed us to the birth center and we were settled in by 10:30 P.M. Mary examined me and I was eight centimeters dilated. Between contractions I would walk out to see Fabio playing with all the neat things JoAnne brought to keep him entertained. She was great with Fabio, even though she said I made her a nervous wreck by walking around at eight centimeters. It did feel good to be able to walk around and not be confined to a bed as in the hospital.

Fabio was so excited and wanted to know and see everything that was going on. He'd come running down the hall to my room every once in a while, ask if the baby had come yet, climb up in bed, and help Lawrence rub my stomach while I was having a contraction. When he saw that the contraction was over (when I stopped breathing funny) he'd go running back to his play things. JoAnne was always right there with him, letting him move about freely, which was exactly what Lawrence and I wanted him to be able to do. When choosing a support person for Fabio, we knew JoAnne was the perfect choice. We wanted someone who not only was loving, affectionate, and fun, but who would also be in tune with Fabio. She fully prepared herself and Fabio by taking the necessary classes offered by the birth center, which we all felt were terrific.

Transition began and my water broke during a very strong contraction. I never experienced this with Fabio, so I was startled. I felt a sort of popping sensation with a gush of very warm water. It seemed to slow down and then there was another quick gush. It was incredible—I really like the feeling. The bed beneath me was soaked and Mary quickly put some clean sheets under me. Then things really started moving.

After much pushing with the help of Lawrence, Mary decided I'd need an episiotomy, so JoAnne quickly took Fabio out while I was being cut, something we decided upon beforehand. They came back in as I started to push again and it didn't take long. At 12:04 A.M., August 4, 1986, tightly squeezing Lawrence's hand and hearing his gentle words of encouragement, I pushed with all I had and out came the baby's head. Fabio looked up at JoAnne with a beaming smile and Mary exclaimed, "It's a girl!" How she knew just by seeing the head was baffling to us, but she was right. One more push and the rest of the baby was delivered, causing Fabio to grin from ear to ear. I finally opened my eyes to see the birth of our beautiful baby girl, Sophia. How wonderful!

Our joy was indescribable. The birth center provided a wonderful setting for the birth of our daughter and offered us choices that were invaluable to us. The choice to have our baby in a warm, homelike environment, the choice to have a small, intimate, family-attended birth, and the choice to have our son present at the birth. Even the choice to decide at the last minute whether or not to let him view the birth. The birth center provided excellent care, excellent facilities, and the result . . . excellence!

Vicki's Story

*Each birth I have attended has been special, but for my husband, Rick, and I, the birth of our daughter Emily was the most special birth of all. As each birth has its own story, ours is no exception. Our story certainly has its share of "Oh, that will **never** happen to me!" That's what makes the telling of it so much fun.*

*Rick's brother was getting married June 23. Not being due until July 7 and knowing that no one **ever** goes before their due date, we looked forward to the gala celebration. I must say it was difficult deciding what to wear to the wedding. When your belly is sticking out to nine months' size and your feet feel like four-by-fours, it's hard to look glamorous. Undaunted, I wore my very best nine months' size dress and as it turned out, I was thankful I had not invested in something fancier.*

We arrived at the bride's parents' home, where the wedding was to take place. We passed through some rooms with lovely oriental rugs and hardwood floors. I'm glad we didn't stop there to chat. We ended up sitting on the patio's wrought iron furniture chatting with two male guests (neither of whom had children). One asked, "When is the baby coming?" and just as he spoke my bag of water broke and water soaked the back of my dress, running down my legs into my shoes. I replied, "I think maybe today" and with that one man began pacing, the other looked stunned, and Rick asked

"Really?" Well, everything really livened up quickly—the word spread like wildfire. It was hard for me to believe it was happening because no one ever breaks their bag in the middle of the day on Long Island at a wedding. I started contracting mildly immediately, which made everyone very nervous, and they were soon on the phone to an obstetrician friend in New York City. We had wanted to stay for the ceremony, since Rick was to participate in it, but we realized very quickly it would not only be foolish but it would have driven everyone else crazy. So, off we went and drove the three and a half hours back home. It was a beautiful, warm summer day and a wonderful drive home knowing that soon our child would be in our arms.

The labor progressed smoothly and I was blessed with an efficient labor. I had ten hours of early labor and then at midnight I went directly into good, strong labor. We arrived at the birth center at 12:45 A.M. It was clear and summer cool, a perfect night for birthing a baby. I've never been one for lots of noise, so it was perfect just having Rick and Anne sitting at my side quietly helping me through the contractions. Little talk, no music, just the work of labor.

I dilated rapidly and by 3:15 A.M. was ready to push. I knew my wide hips would come in handy someday. I only had to push sixteen minutes before Emily was helped into this world by Anne and Rick. We welcomed her with our cries of joy as she laid on my abdomen taking in her new world. She was peaceful and content.

Many have asked—did you learn anything from the experience? I can honestly say that I learned even more personally why I love midwifery. Everyone needs someone by their side in labor besides their family. Someone who has been at many births and has the perspective and expertise that comes from attending many women. There is a reassurance that comes from being individually cared for that then allows the family to get on with the business of having their baby. As so many others have said—I couldn't have done it without my husband and my midwife.

Debbie's Story

When I became pregnant, my gynecologist became my obstetrician. I never gave a thought to changing doctors. In preparing for childbirth, I read all the books I could find. During my fourth month, I read about the Bradley method of natural childbirth and was convinced of the rightness of the many things I wanted my birth to be (including detailed breathing, relaxing, and massaging exercises we could practice).

After reading this book, however, we were concerned that the probability of having a completely natural birth at the hospital was lower than at a birth center or home birth. In discussing our concerns with my obstetrician we learned that he was required to practice within the guidelines of the American School of Obstetrics and within the hospital rules; that various residents and nurses would be looking after me in the hospital as the shifts changed every eight hours; that midwives could not be "hired" as nurses in the hospital; and that the hospital had only one "birthing room" which had a bathroom in it. After our discussion my obstetrician suggested that we talk with the midwives at the birth center. I was eight months pregnant at the time and had not heard of the birth center until that moment. That suggestion was the best thing that happened to us during the pregnancy.

By that point, we had already attended the hospital's prenatal classes. We were disappointed that so much time was spent discussing medicated births and very little was spent on natural births. We were not interested in the detailed discussions on C-sections, episiotomies, and the various drugs available at various stages of labor. Looking around the class one evening, I remember thinking how sad it was that probably two out of the ten of us would have C-sections. Even the class members seemed timid and scared, rather than excited and ready for childbirth.

Putting all of these things together, we decided to switch in my ninth month to the birth center. I had had a "normal" pregnancy that far and I was hoping for a "normal" delivery. For us, the birth center was the lower-risk option.

From that point on, everything that happened just reassured us that we had made the right decision. The people we met in classes were confident and excited and the classes focused on natural childbirth. All the midwives were knowledgeable, cheerful, and helpful.

My labor began at 12:15 A.M. on June 1, when my water broke in bed. We were able to return to sleep, as contractions did not begin until 6:30 A.M. While I labored at home my labor followed this pattern: 6:30 to 10:00—erratic contractions, 7 to 15 minutes apart; 10:00 to 11:00—easy contractions, 5 to 7 minutes apart; 11:00 to 1:00—stronger contractions, 3 to 5 minutes apart; 1:00 to 3:00—strong contractions, 2 to 3 minutes apart. I was able to stand or sit during all of these contractions. They felt like stomach pains, as if I had eaten something which did not agree with me. I also had a bad case of diarrhea all morning. Going to the bathroom was far more painful than the contractions!

We phoned the birth center at 8:00 A.M. and again at 1:00 P.M. We were asked to come in around 3:00 P.M., which we did. The car ride was absolutely awful. Both accelerating and decelerating made the contractions very strong. I found a "comfortable" position on my side, curled up in a ball.

I was four centimeters dilated when we arrived. Once there, I walked around upstairs for as along as I could. My contractions were 1-1/2 to 2 minutes apart and very strong. I was able to breathe through them normally, but not without difficulty. Because of the diarrhea, I chose to have an enema. Not only did it make that pain go away, but I knew I would not have to go again before the baby was born! It also may have sped up my labor.

By 4:30 the contractions were very strong and I chose to lie down. I do not remember the contractions as "painful," until I began to get the "combination" contractions (where at the peak of a first-stage contraction comes a second stage or pushing contraction). This happened around 5:30 and from that point on, I had to blow and breathe very fast to avoid grunting (pushing) and letting the contraction get away from me. This transition phase was tough, but not unbearable. I went from six centimeters to 10 centimeters between 4:30 and 6:30. Then I was told I could give in to the pushing contractions.

During the next hour, whenever a contraction came, I pushed with my whole body. My face was beet red, my neck veins were bulging, my arms were very tense. I did not realize how much less effective this full-body pushing was until an hour went by and the baby had not moved much. It hurt so much to push correctly that I was trying to avoid pushing in that way. I was very disappointed in myself. Someone suggested that I readjust my attitude. Truthfully I was not prepared for the discomfort and effort of pushing. I thought pushing would be a "relief." For me, it was not. Around 7:30 I finally got mad enough to begin pushing more where the baby was and pushing into the hurt.

I remember wondering if I would ever make any progress, as I did not feel any differently at 8:00 than I had at 6:30. Was I surprised when asked to look down . . . there was half of the baby's head! No wonder it was so uncomfortable! Seeing the head gave me a second wind. I should have looked in a mirror sooner! It took a few more pushes to birth the head, at which time the midwives cleared the mucus and checked for the cord. About thirty seconds later, I was asked to push again. The baby had one hand tucked up under its chin, which made it harder to clear the shoulders. About a minute later, the shoulders popped out and I was asked to take my baby and pull it the rest of the way out. What a surprise!! I pulled her out and laid her on my chest. It was 8:17 P.M.

What a wonderful moment! I'll never forget it.

I held her for a long time while she was wiped off and admired by my husband and me. She finally cried, after what seemed like a long time. I held her while the midwives assisted with the birth of the placenta. This was a slightly painful process. I held her while I received a few sutures (due primarily to the position of her hand under her chin). I fed her soon after that. What an amazing sucking reflex babies have! She seemed to be starving!

The sentiments expressed in these birth stories are expressed over and over again by birth center clients. Women talk about the caring and support offered by the nurse-midwives. They talk about the comfortable atmosphere of the birth center and the attachment they feel to the place itself. Mostly, women talk about feeling empowered by the experience of giving birth under the supportive circumstances which the birth center provides.

Over the course of my research I have spoken with only a handful of women who have described negative aspects of their birth center experience. In only one of those cases did the woman opt to leave the birth center and seek the services of a physician for the remainder of her pregnancy. In the other cases the dissatisfaction stemmed from a difficult relationship with a particular midwife or with one of the backup physicians. While these women did not leave the birth center, they did express mixed feelings about their experience there.

The newsletter in which the birth stories appeared has been published off and on over the years by birth center clients and supporters. In addition to birth stories, the newsletter has carried a variety of information that is useful to expectant parents and to parents of young children. One issue, for example, focused on circumcision. It contained some basic information on the procedure as well as a variety of perspectives on circumcision from birth center clients, both mothers and fathers. Another issue focused on concerns about the body and sexuality which often surface for women during pregnancy and following birth. Birth center clients talked about the positive experiences they had had as well as some of the difficulties they had experienced. One woman wrote about the difficulty of maintaining a sexual relationship with one's partner following the birth of a child. She talked about her own experience with this issue and offered some insight into the changing relationships between partners once children are part of the picture. Other women wrote on the benefits of swimming and tai chi to keep the body toned and promote emotional well-being. Still others wrote about societal images of women's bodies which deny the realities of women's lives.

The newsletter has also been used to keep supporters up to date on issues of importance to the birth center. When a malpractice insurance crisis threatened the birth center, the newsletter was used to explain the nature of the problem and to suggest directions for political action.

The newsletter has served as an important vehicle of communication among birth center clients, many of whom stay involved with the center long after their childbearing experiences. It is a vehicle which clients use to express their positive feelings about the birth center. It is also a way for information and ideas to be exchanged.

DISCUSSION

The birth center has created a birth setting with extremely positive results for the clients it serves. The needs and concerns of the pregnant woman are the focus of care at the center. The nurse-midwives seek to empower women by providing them with the information they need to make decisions about their own pregnancy, labor, and delivery and by creating an environment in which women have much more control over their experience than they do in a hospital setting. The relationship between nurse-midwives and clients is built on equality, trust, and a shared belief that childbirth is a unique experience for each woman.

For the most part the women who come to the birth center are not women who would have chosen home birth, at least in the state which I studied. Many women felt a sense of security at the birth center which home birth did not provide for them. Most important, clients develop a strong sense of attachment to the nurse-midwives, the nurses, and the center itself. The birth center is not home, nor is it simply another institutional alternative to the hospital. The birth center represents a community of women and families who view the center as a place where birth can be experienced to the fullest and where women are left with a strong sense of their own ability to nurture life and give birth.

The establishment of a birth center has provided an alternative within the context of the medical model of birthing. Arney's (1982) arguments on alternatives to the medical model are particularly relevant here. Arney maintains that most alternatives are not alternatives in any true sense since they all fall within the limits of discourse established by the medical establishment. While the birth center does create an environment that seeks to empower women, it is clear that dominant practices are embedded in institutions with a range of powers that constrain the emergence of birthing settings and practices which challenge the medical model.

The chapter which follows analyzes the constraints imposed by the medical model and considers the extent to which the birth center has been able to operate independently of the medical model. To the extent that the center has operated independently, how vulnerable is it to reassertion of dominance by the medical model?

8

The Birth Center
and the Medical Model:
Accommodation and Resistance

The continued existence of the birth center rests upon maintaining established relationships with institutions that are embedded in the medical model of childbirth. While the birth center and the medical model are interrelated, their relationship is asymmetrical, with the balance of power resting with the medical-legal establishment. The institutions associated with the medical model have responded to the birth center by offering a somewhat wider array of choices to birthing women. In effect, birthing practices have expanded through the medical model's response to the birth center. When the birth center was in the early planning stage, for example, the medical center responded by opening a birthing room. Birthing rooms resemble bedrooms in appearance and lack the harshness of a standard labor room. Low-risk women who expect no complications with their delivery are eligible to use a birthing room. According to surveys conducted by the medical center over the first two years of operation of the birthing room, those who used it liked it very much. Once the birth center was established, the medical center also changed its policy on sibling visitation, allowing siblings to visit immediately following birth. While the new policy was originally intended for and used by women giving birth in the birthing room, sibling visitation is now accepted policy for all women giving birth at the medical center. Children can visit with their mothers shortly after birth and can get to see their new sister or brother. The medical center has recently opened a new maternity wing with combined labor-delivery-recovery rooms. The practice of combining the labor, delivery, and recovery rooms means that women do not have to be moved from one room to another while they are in active labor or immediately after birth. Rooms such as these are becoming more common as hospitals build new maternity facilities or renovate old ones.

At the same time, the existence of the birth center is, to a large extent, dependent upon recognition and support by dominant institutions. While the birth center has been open and functioning for over twelve years, its operation has been markedly affected by the links which it has to the medical model. The degree to which the birth center is consistent with the medical model has helped the center to become established and to remain open but there are also costs associated with operating within this framework. Some of those costs include (1) a lack of wider linkages with those active around women's and social equity issues, (2) problems with third-party reimbursement, (3) difficulties with malpractice insurance, (4) opposition to the center from the medical establishment, and (5) a dwindling client base.

LACK OF WIDER LINKAGES

For most of the birth center's history those involved with the birth center have not networked with groups which might be supportive of the center but which might generate opposition from the establishment, such as feminist groups. The goal of those involved with the center has been to provide a safe, woman-centered option for birthing women. While this is certainly an important goal and one which has led to the availability of a valuable childbirth alternative in the area, it is also a very narrow goal. It does not tie the birth center to any larger feminist agenda concerning women's reproductive rights or women's rights more generally. There is an active feminist community in the area organized around abortion rights, curbing domestic violence and sexual assault, and improving material conditions for women. Some birth center clients and supporters share these concerns and identify themselves as feminists. Others, however, reject feminism and are strongly antichoice. This presents a dilemma in terms of shaping broad-based political support for the birth center.

THIRD-PARTY REIMBURSEMENT

Both third-party reimbursement and malpractice insurance are essential for the operation of the birth center. Without third-party reimbursement, many people would be financially unable to choose the birth center over traditional obstetric care. Without malpractice insurance, the nurse-midwives as well as their backup physicians would be without financial protection in the event of a lawsuit.

When the birth center solidified its plans to open, Blue Cross/Blue Shield in the state drew up criteria for evaluating birth centers. The purpose of the criteria, according to a spokesperson for Blue Cross/Blue Shield, is to insure that subscribers receive quality care. Reflecting state law, the criteria require that nurse-midwives working at free-standing birth centers have a written agreement with at least one obstetrician and one pediatrician. The reason for this requirement is to insure that there is physician involvement in developing policies and procedures for the center. Physicians are not required to be on site for births but must be available for consultation and backup. Blue Cross/Blue Shield also requires that birth centers file for a certificate of need with the state. Once a birth center demonstrates that it can meet these criteria, Blue Cross/Blue Shield will enter into negotiations with it regarding reimbursement.

When the birth center opened there was no law in the state which mandated third-party reimbursement for nurse-midwives. Initially, however, things generally went smoothly with third-party payers, particularly with Blue Cross/Blue Shield. One important factor which contributed to this was that the person who negotiated contracts between providers and subscribers for Blue Cross/Blue Shield had two children born at the birth center. Also, the fact that birth center births cost roughly half of a routine vaginal delivery in the hospital made them an attractive option.

During the summer of 1985 problems began to develop with insurance claims filed by the center. Companies began to insist that before claims could be processed they needed certain information about the center (such as whether the center had a physician as medical director) and documentation, such as a copy of the center's license. In addition, a couple of large employers in the area, including the local medical center, refused to include birth center services among their insurance benefits. It became clear that mandated third-party reimbursement was important to the continued operation of the center. Not only were the problems with reimbursement discouraging some potential birth center clients, they were also contributing to staffing problems at the center. When nurse-midwives had a choice they were going to states which had mandated coverage because it made their employment more secure.

The nurse-midwives at the center became involved in an effort to get legislation passed which would mandate third-party reimbursement for nurse-midwives. This legislation was discussed at a meeting in February 1988 of the Women's Legislative Roundtable, a group made up of representatives from area women's organizations, including the state chapter of the National Organization for Women (NOW), the state commission for women, the YWCA, and others. The roundtable holds regular meetings, which are open to the public, to discuss potential or proposed legislation and its impact on women. The group which met to discuss nurse-midwifery legislation included about thirty people, among them representatives from the groups mentioned above, a class of students from a nearby university, two representatives from the state legislature, representatives from the press, and a few former birth center clients.

Eunice K. Ernst, then director of the National Association of Childbearing Centers (NACC), gave a presentation on dominant childbirth practices and the alternative which birth centers and nurse-midwives offer. She was quite outspoken in her criticisms of physicians and dominant practices, arguing that the standard obstetric care which most women receive is tantamount to abuse. She also talked about the cost of childbirth and rising health care costs generally and said that birth centers provide a cost-effective alternative to hospital birth. Her presentation was more radical in both style and content than that of Anne Watson, who directs the center.

Anne gave a presentation illustrated by slides of the center itself and of women laboring and giving birth at the center. She argued that legislation which mandates third-party reimbursement for nurse-midwives was necessary if the birth center was to survive. She reported that she was having trouble hiring nurse-midwives to work at the center because of the precarious nature of employment for nurse-midwives in the state. Getting such legislation passed required support from those groups active around women's issues in the state, and Anne appealed to them. The person who was chair of NOW's (state chapter) family law task force at the time is a former birth center client, and she organized people to work on drafting the legislation and sought legislative sponsors.

Initially this appeal for support from women's organizations, particularly NOW, appeared to be a significant departure for Anne Watson and others involved with the birth center. If one looks at how the issue was framed and presented, however, it is not at all clear that this is the case. At the roundtable meeting, a summary of the problem was presented by the chair of NOW's family law task force. She argued that it was important to support legislation which would help keep nurse-midwives in business for three main reasons:

1. The state has a very high infant mortality rate, and the care which nurse-midwives provide could help to lower that rate.

2. Nurse-midwifery care is cost-effective; birth center costs are roughly half those for standard obstetrical care and hospital delivery.

3. Nurse-midwives and the care they provide contribute to the quality of life for the individuals they service.

The appeal made to the public for support and the appeal to the legislature had nothing to do with women's rights but instead focused on dimensions of the dominant political economy.

Following the meeting I spoke with the head of NOW's family law task force, who said that although NOW supported this legislation and helped organize the effort to see it passed, they took all their direction on the issue from Anne Watson. Anne preferred not to present the issue as a feminist one because doing so would not be acceptable to many of those in power. Nevertheless, the appeal to women's organizations for any degree of support was a step beyond the narrow bounds previously maintained by birth center supporters.

Anne Watson wrote personally to every member of the state legislature to explain the significance of this legislation for nurse-midwives. She stressed the important contributions which nurse-midwives make to the health care of women and babies in the state. Birth center supporters drew up a phone tree which divided birth center clients into representative and senatorial districts and called clients to request that they contact their legislators about the bill. So many clients wrote about the bill that the chair of the state's Health and Human Services Committee at the time commented on the volume of mail he had received. Efforts to pass legislation mandating third-party reimbursement for nurse-midwives were successful: the bill was signed into law in July 1988. The effort gave nurse-midwives and the birth center much more public visibility than they had had before. It succeeded in generating strong support among some members of the state legislature who could be called upon again if the need arose. Still, the appeal for support from outside groups was specific to the particular issue of mandated third-party reimbursement. There was no effort to build a more broadly based coalition of citizen support that might provide more general support for nurse-midwifery and for the birth center.

MALPRACTICE INSURANCE

During the center's initial years of operation there were no problems with malpractice insurance. Both the nurse-midwives and the center itself were covered at a nominal cost. In 1985, however, the malpractice situation drastically changed. Many providers of medical malpractice insurance began to cancel policies for health care providers.

In June 1985, Mutual Fire Marine and Inland Insurance Company of Philadelphia announced that it would not renew any medical malpractice policies after July 3, 1985. Mutual Fire Marine and Inland provided coverage for about one-half of all the nurse-midwives in the country. Richard Guilfoyle, president of the company, said that they insured 1,289 nurse-midwives for $1 million each, for a total risk of roughly $1.2 billion. According to Guilfoyle, the upheaval over the question of medical malpractice stemmed from increases in the size of awards and in the number of lawsuits between 1980 and 1985. He claimed that between 1980 and 1985, insurance companies had actually lost money because of the size of jury awards in malpractice cases.

While nurse-midwives were charged lower rates than obstetricians or other physicians for the purposes of coverage, they all came under the same category of medical malpractice. When Mutual Fire Marine and Inland made the decision to drop all its medical malpractice coverage, nurse-midwives were dropped along with physicians, despite the fact that nurse-midwives are rarely sued. At the time, about 6 percent of nurse-midwives had been sued, whereas 66.9 percent of obstetricians had been sued at least once.

While the public announcement about the insurance cancellation did not come until June 1985, the nurse-midwives at the birth center had been informed in December 1984 that their malpractice coverage as well as coverage for the center itself would not be renewed. Anne Watson decided to work on a solution to this problem behind the scenes with a small group of people. The first steps taken had to do with changing the institutional structure of the birth center. Early in 1985, the name of the center was changed. In April, a foundation was formed for the purpose of supporting and educating the public about nurse-midwifery and childbirth alternatives in the state. The foundation was the successor to the original nonprofit community board of directors which owned and operated the center. Anne Watson bought out the birth center's assets and converted the center to a for-profit organization. All of the assets of the nonprofit organization were transferred to the foundation. This move legally separated the foundation and its assets from the birth center, protecting those assets in the event of any suits against the center or the nurse-midwives. The disbanding of the community board of directors protected those individuals from lawsuits brought against the center's nurse-midwives.

In early 1985, the cancellation of malpractice coverage was viewed as a problem by the nurse-midwives, but not as an insurmountable one. At that point they felt that they would have to search for a new source of coverage and that new coverage would be considerably more expensive than what they had previously paid. They did not think that coverage would not be available to them even at increased cost. By the time of the public announcement in June, however, it was clear to those closely involved with the center that the problem was much more serious than they had originally thought.

According to the National Association of Childbearing Centers, six birth centers had already closed by June 1985, due to lack of insurance coverage. The American College of Nurse-Midwives was looking for some blanket solution to the problem and had already talked with the Federal Trade

Commission (FTC) about possible action over the insurance issue on the grounds of restraint of trade. Meanwhile, nurse-midwives were being encouraged to seek solutions in individual states. It was at this point that Anne decided to involve a wider network of people in searching for a solution to the malpractice problem.

A task force of concerned birth center clients was formed, and it held its initial meeting on August 20, 1985. At that meeting Anne explained the birth center's insurance situation. The insurance for the center itself had expired on August 10, and Anne's individual coverage was due to expire on October 1. She said that while she was willing to practice without insurance, she could not do so because this would put the center's backup physicians in jeopardy.

The job of the task force was to determine a number of possible routes to obtaining malpractice insurance and insuring the survival of the center. The options ranged from self-insurance for nurse-midwives to state and national legislation that would guarantee some type of insurance for nurse-midwives. The consensus of the group was that while national and state laws could supply long-term solutions, time was short and a more expedient plan was necessary. It was decided that as many avenues as possible should be pursued, including the following:

1. meeting with those in charge of health benefits for the large local employers, since they had included the birth center's services in the insurance package for their employees and had an interest in the center's survival

2. meeting with the state insurance commissioner

3. sending a letter to the FTC notifying them that some type of coercion possibly was taking place against insurance companies that were insuring nurse-midwives

4. supplying those on the birth center's mailing list with postcards to send to the insurance commissioner and state representatives urging that something be done about the problem

Some members of the task force wanted to do nothing to alienate any political officials. The group should not come across as "demanding" action on this issue but rather as "requesting" that something be done. Although some members of the group disagreed with this "soft-touch" approach, they were in a minority. The majority were politically moderate, and their approach to the malpractice issue was characterized by a fear of being perceived as "rocking the boat." Yet groups in other nearby states were successful in gaining insurance during this period by making their demands explicit through marches, rallies, telegrams, and phone calls. While the task force was aware of the success of stronger tactics, many members of the group were opposed to using similar methods in their particular state.

By September 1985, members of the task force had visited the governor, the insurance commissioner, a congressional representative, and a senator. They were also in the process of investigating somewhat creative solutions, such as becoming a branch of a birth center in a nearby state since that center was insured. Time was quickly running out, however, and no obvious solutions were available.

Anne Watson began looking into the possibility of obtaining practicing privileges at a local hospital for herself and the other nurse-midwives at the center. In the event that malpractice insurance for the center could not be located, clients could give birth at this hospital. If the nurse-midwives had practicing privileges there, they would be protected by the hospital's malpractice coverage. Just before Anne approached the hospital, a letter was sent to area physicians urging them to inform the hospital that they would boycott the hospital if privileges were granted to nurse-midwives. When Anne spoke with the director of the hospital, she told him she knew about the letter. She was told that nurse-midwives would only fit in under the category of physician's assistant and, therefore, would have to practice under the supervision of a physician. Following the meeting Anne Watson informed the director in writing that physician's assistant was not an appropriate category for nurse-midwives and that the hospital needed to develop guidelines for nurse-midwifery practice. No further developments occurred on the issue of practicing privileges for nurse-midwives at that point. In 1992, however, the same hospital did grant practicing privileges to a local nurse-midwife who had previously worked at the birth center. Nurse-midwives also have practicing privileges in another county in the state, where they staff public health clinics and attend more than seven hundred births per year. The state's largest newspaper credits the work of nurse-midwives for the county's low infant mortality rate. As of 1992, the rate for that county was 9.8 deaths per 1,000 births, while the state as a whole had an infant mortality rate of 11.6 for the same year, higher than the overall U.S. rate. The county where the birth center is located had a rate of 12.6.

Throughout 1985, the birth center had been undergoing renovation. An open house had been scheduled for October 6 to celebrate completion of the renovation. When no insurance had been located by mid-September, it was decided that the open house should be postponed until late October. At that point many birth center supporters were afraid that by October there would be no cause for celebration if some source of insurance could not be located.

Despite the ongoing insurance problem, plans continued for the October 20, 1985, open house at the birth center. Throughout September representatives from the center were working closely with the insurance commissioner to locate coverage. The open house was held on October 20 as scheduled. The insurance commissioner attended the event and announced that an insurance company based in a nearby state had agreed to insure the nurse-midwives at the center. Rates for this new coverage were markedly higher than those previously paid; they ranged from $2,842 for $300,000 worth of coverage to $5,827 for up to $3 million in coverage. Previously, the center's midwives had paid $840 for up to $3 million in coverage. At the time the nurse-midwives at the center were earning about $25,000 per year, so the new rates accounted for a large percentage of their yearly income.

This new solution proved to be very short-lived. The company which had agreed to provide coverage was a physicians' insurance company. Shortly after it began insuring the birth center, it started putting pressure on the nurse-midwives to change their routine practices of attending births at the center and providing routine physical examinations. Because these demands were unacceptable, it became clear that the nurse-midwives had to either locate another source of malpractice coverage or close the center. The insurance commissioner once again helped, this time by convincing a Swedish company based in New York to provide $250,000 of malpractice protection for the nurse-midwives at the center.

In the meantime, lobbying efforts by the American College of Nurse-Midwives proved successful at the national level. Despite opposition from the insurance lobby, Congress passed amendments to the Risk Retention Act in early 1986 which allow small groups to incorporate for the purposes of purchasing insurance. A group of nurse-midwives from across the country incorporated in a single state in order to be able to buy insurance in that state. Immediately following passage of the legislation, a consortium of six insurance companies came forward and offered malpractice coverage to nurse-midwives. Each of the six companies insures some of the nurse-midwives in order to divide the risk. The total amount of coverage carried by each nurse-midwife is $250,000. Nurse-midwives and other medical practitioners are now being advised by insurance companies to carry less insurance. The companies argue that the amount of insurance coverage contributes to the size of suits being brought against practitioners.

The malpractice insurance crisis experienced by the nurse-midwives is an indication of the center's vulnerability. Nurse-midwives lost malpractice coverage because they were categorized as health care providers along with physicians, despite the fact that nurse-midwives pose very little financial risk. Although physicians were not responsible for the loss of malpractice insurance by nurse-midwives in the state, they exacerbated the situation by threatening to boycott a local hospital if practicing privileges were granted there to nurse-midwives.

At the same time that the malpractice insurance crisis demonstrates the center's vulnerability, however, it also points to some significant sources of support. The role of the insurance commissioner in helping the center to obtain insurance coverage is particularly important to note. There is no indication that the commissioner had any particular commitment to childbirth alternatives, but his actions on the malpractice insurance issue provided another buffer between the center and the considerable power of physicians in the area. The center may not have survived without the interim solutions for which the commissioner was responsible.

Throughout the malpractice insurance crisis, the center was tied to a network of individuals and groups seeking a solution to the insurance problem. The strength of this network, which included the National Association of Childbearing Centers, the American Nursing Association, and the American College of Nurse-Midwives, was enough to draw national attention to the problem and to encourage passage of the Risk Retention Act of 1986.

Malpractice insurance continues to be a problem for the center. At the present time there are too few clients at the center to support two full-time nurse-midwives. The malpractice insurance coverage held by the center will not cover part-time workers. As mentioned in an earlier chapter, it is hoped that insurance currently available for birth centers and their full-time staff members will soon be extended to part-time staff as well. Such a policy would be important for this birth center or any other which has part-time employees.

OPPOSITION FROM THE BOARD OF MEDICINE

Along with the malpractice insurance problem, the birth center began experiencing conflicts with the state board of medicine in January 1985. The board had been putting pressure on the center's backup physicians by maintaining that the nurse-midwives needed special clearance by the board in order to provide such routine services as attending births, administering any drugs, and inserting intrauterine devices (IUDs) for contraception. Expressing support for the center and a desire to be as helpful as possible, the physicians asked the board to let them know what they could do to help in this situation. There was no immediate response from the board of medicine.

At the annual meeting of the American Medical Association (AMA) held in Honolulu in December 1984, the house of delegates voted in support of a resolution requiring the development of a strategy to fight incursions into medical practice by nonphysician practitioners including nurse-midwives, podiatrists, nurse-practitioners, physician's assistants, psychologists, nurse-anesthetists, and optometrists. The physicians were particularly opposed to new legislation extending medical practice rights, including prescribing privileges, independent practice, and mandated third-party reimbursement, to these practitioners.

While the center had been functioning relatively free of harassment for three years, it started to appear as though a whole new set of obstacles were being put in its path. Obtaining malpractice insurance emerged as a central problem which nearly forced the center to close. The AMA resolution, an obvious indication that physicians intended to maintain their opposition to nonphysician practitioners, was, of course, a reaction to the whole crop of establishments that had been gaining some autonomy since the late 1970s, including birth centers, surgi-centers, and the private practices of nurse-practitioners. The physicians may have feared competition. The number of doctors in private practice in the United States increased dramatically between 1960 and 1980 (Starr, 1982). At the same time there has been a slowdown in population growth. Starr argues, however, that whether this will result in a surplus of doctors has more to do with politics than with numbers. Demand will be affected by national health legislation and changes in public and private health insurance. He also states, "The demand for doctors' services might also be reduced by the incursions of related professionals and paramedical workers; or increased, if those alternatives are cut off by restrictive licensing and reimbursement practices" (1982, p. 422).

The entire time the center has been in operation, physicians in the area have flexed their muscles in various ways to try to keep the center from operating or to limit the scope and autonomy of nurse-midwives. They have never been completely successful, but they have been able to place several stumbling blocks in the way of the nurse-midwives. This demonstrates the vulnerability of the birth center to the medical establishment. Efforts to overcome these various barriers require time and effort which could be spent on caregiving and other activities of more benefit to individuals and the community.

At the present time, everything relating to health care in our society is in a state of flux. There are some indications that nonphysician practitioners such as nurses and nurse-midwives might be given a larger and more autonomous role in the evolving structure. New legislation in many states is giving advanced practice nurses privileges to diagnose illness and prescribe medication that they did not have before. On the other hand, the structure of health care is becoming more bureaucratized and centralized. Insurance companies and large hospitals are expanding their role in the organization and provision of health care. Although birth centers will almost certainly be affected, it is too soon to tell what all of the effects will be.

DWINDLING CLIENT BASE

The number of birth center clients peaked in the late 1980s and then began dropping until 1992. Currently there are between 130 and 135 births per year. This number has been stable for the past couple of years but there is a serious concern about how to increase the number of women who come to the birth center for pregnancy and birth.

Anne attributes some of the drop-off in birth center clients to an increased use of epidural anesthesia at the local medical center. According to Anne, about 70 percent of women giving birth at the medical center receive epidurals. She believes that the popularity of this anesthesia and a more general fear of giving birth outside the hospital make women reluctant to come to the birth center.

One of the tasks for Anne and her supporters over the years has been to think of ways to inform the public about the existence of the birth center and to encourage birthing women to consider this location for giving birth. A variety of efforts have been made, including radio and television spots, magazine ads, and public forums, but they have met with minimal success. Some people come to the center as a result of these outreach attempts but not many. Instead, word-of-mouth referrals account for 97 percent of the center's clients. In addition, there are people in the community who do not know the center exists despite the fact that it has been in operation for twelve years.

Anne has said that the current size of the client base raises some serious problems. The birth center can now cover its costs, but it would not be able to do so if the client base got much smaller. Nor can a client base of the current size support two full-time nurse-midwives. This in turn creates additional problems. First of all, as mentioned earlier, the current malpractice policy which the center carries will not cover part-time employees. Second, the lack of another full-time nurse-midwife creates an enormous burden for Anne, who not only works in an administrative capacity as director of the center but also covers most of the clinic hours, seeing clients for prenatal and well-woman care. In addition, she is on call most of the time for births.

One of the main sources of support for the birth center since 1985 has come from the nonprofit foundation board which was formed at the time of the malpractice crisis. The assets of the birth center were transferred to the foundation which holds the funds in trust. A small amount of money is kept in a cash account, but the bulk of the money has been used to purchase certificates of deposit. The money generates about five thousand dollars per year in interest, which is used to pay for various projects which the board sponsors. The foundation also conducts an annual campaign during which funds are solicited from current and former clients. The most recent fundraising effort raised about two thousand dollars. Together with the interest on the foundation accounts, the funds make it possible for projects to be carried out without spending any of the principal. To meet its stated purpose of providing public education about nurse-midwifery, the board engages in a number of activities. It conducts public forums where invited speakers talk about nurse-midwifery. Penny Armstrong, author of *A Midwife's Tale* and *Wise Birth*, has given two public lectures on behalf of the foundation board. The board also does presentations on nurse-midwifery and birth centers for local high schools and colleges. Occasionally the board participates in health fairs and baby fairs, where booths are set up with information about nurse-midwifery and birth centers. For a number of years the foundation has provided scholarship money to a nurse-midwifery student who is close to completing her education. Priority is given to nurse-midwives who plan to practice in the area in which the birth center is located. Despite this priority, however, no one who has received this scholarship has ever returned to the birth center to practice. The foundation board also assists a local program which provides prenatal care to low-income women. Most recently, the board purchased a videocassette player and monitor for this program to be used for educational tapes. The board also provided some breastfeeding tapes in Spanish, since many of the clients of the program are Spanish speaking.

At any one time about ten individuals or couples sit on the foundation board. Couples receive only one vote. Since 1985 there has been some turnover in board members, but most of the current members have served for several years. All but one of them have had children born at the birth center. One board member has had two home births. Many board members come to the center for well-woman care.

As might be expected, board members have distinctly different personalities and personal styles. Beyond this, however, they have some differing reasons for being interested in the issues of nurse-midwifery generally and of birth centers in particular. Some board members are interested in alternative approaches to health and well-being. Two members belong to a homeopathy study group and use a homeopath as their primary source of advice regarding their own health and the health of their families. A number of board members visit a chiropractor on a regular basis.

For other board members, politics serves as the motivating force for their activism around the birth center. Feminist in their approach, they see the issue of birthing as part of the larger agenda of reproductive rights for women.

In contrast, until recently one board member was a self-identified funda-
mentalist Christian who was strongly opposed to abortion. She had been a
practicing nurse-midwife before her children were born and continued to be
involved in midwifery education. This member left the board when she
moved out of the area. She had been on the board for a number of years before
leaving, serving as president for some of her tenure.

I do not mean to suggest that the board is made up entirely of people with
distinctly different approaches and agendas. Not all board members are easy
to categorize, and sometimes a board member's approach reflects a variety of
concerns. Someone might be interested in homeopathy and at the same time
be a strong feminist who is politically motivated. For the most part, however,
board members work together well, enjoy each other's company, and share a
deep commitment to the birth center and to Anne. But as a rule broader
political issues are not discussed.

In addition to its stated purpose of providing public education about
midwifery, the board is also very concerned about the continued existence of
the birth center. The foundation board is largely an offshoot of the birth
center, and board members have a direct interest in seeing the center survive.
Their reasons are not strictly personal. This birth center is the only one in
the state. Lay midwifery is illegal; lay midwives do come from out of state to
attend home births, but there are only a small number of home births in the
state each year. If the birth center were to close, childbirth options in the state
would be seriously limited. Some people who now seek out the birth center
would arrange to give birth at home. For many women, however, the birth
center is a radical departure from the typical hospital birth. Most women who
come to the birth center would have their babies in the hospital if the birth
center did not exist.

Although the board has no official connection to the birth center, keeping
the center open has been an ongoing concern. The uncertainty of the birth
center's future makes it difficult for the board to establish a clear direction
for itself. Members are struggling with the question of what will happen to
the birth center and to the board when Anne retires, which is likely to happen
within the next two years. Over the years, the board has discussed the
possibility of buying and running the birth center when Anne leaves, but it
is questionable whether it has the resources to buy and run the birth center.
It is also unclear whether anyone else will buy the practice, particularly if the
client base stays at its current rate or declines.

One of the small local hospitals has been interested in taking over the birth
center for the past several years. They have approached Anne on several
occasions with an offer to buy the practice and the building. They have said
that the nurse-midwives could continue to practice at the birth center but

would not have practicing privileges at the hospital. Anne discussed this option with the foundation board, whose members distrusted the offer. They feared that practice at the birth center would change and that the hospital was really more interested in the building than in the practice. The board members felt that as long as the birth center can survive on its own, Anne should reject the hospital's offer.

At this point, a major concern of the foundation board is using their public education efforts to increase the client base of the birth center. Several strategies have been proposed. The board is looking into hiring a professional marketing analyst and into putting together some public service announcements about nurse-midwifery to increase public awareness. They are also hoping to strengthen their presentations by including not only positive information about birth centers but also negative information about some routine hospital procedures such as epidurals and Cesarean sections. It is the board's plan to reach a wider audience with these presentations by doing lunch time workshops for corporations and organizations. Although there are also plans to strengthen ties to other health-oriented groups in the area, board members have reservations about working with organizations which provide abortion services because birth center clients disagree on the issue of abortion. Finally, board members strongly believe that it is necessary to tap more effectively the resource of the current clientele. Since 97 percent of the referrals to the birth center are by word of mouth, birth center clients need to be encouraged to spread the word about the birth center. To this end, the board hopes that fliers about the birth center can be included in the packets which new parents take home when they leave the center. These strategies represent a somewhat broader approach than the foundation board has ever taken before. Whether they will be successful in increasing the client base remains to be seen.

DISCUSSION

The birth center has been in existence for twelve years. During that time over 1,600 births have occurred at the center, and almost all of the women who have given birth there have reported positive experiences.

It is the case, however, that this birth center, and free-standing birth centers more generally, are in many ways tied to the medical model. These ties create constraints for nurse-midwives practicing in birth centers and make birth centers vulnerable to the power of dominant medical-legal institutions and practices.

This chapter discussed some of the ways in which the medical model shapes the context in which the birth center operates. Over the years problems have emerged with third-party reimbursement, malpractice insurance, and opposition from physicians. Other problems have been related to the shrinking size of the client base. The medical model of birth with its reliance on technology and painkilling drugs is part of our cultural consciousness. Deciding to have a baby at the birth center requires a rejection of the culture's most basic beliefs about birth. It seems that more women were willing to do that in the 1980s than they are in the 1990s, at least in the area where this center is located. The fact that the number of birth centers in existence nationwide has declined since the late 1980s indicates that this trend may be general rather than local.

The birth center faces a difficult dilemma. On the one hand, the center challenges patterns of expertise, technological dependence, and male-dominated practice characteristic of the medical model. On the other hand, it is itself embedded in and requires support from the institutional, financial, and cultural relations of the medical model. The history of this birth center demonstrates the vulnerability of this position. The question which remains is whether it is possible to develop political circumstances which would decrease the center's vulnerability or whether these problems are inherent within the concept of the free-standing birth center.

9

Reappropriating Birth

In this book I have discussed relationships among technology, authority, and gender as they shape dominant childbirth practices and woman-centered challenges to these practices. I have explored how technology is appropriated by dominant institutions to construct birth as both an ideology and as an instrumental practice that supports the domination of women.

Woman-centered facilities, such as free-standing birth centers, stand in partial opposition to this technocratic, medical model. A critical tension arises between these two that leads to some innovations in dominant birthing practices, on the one hand, and accommodations to the medical model by those who challenge it, on the other.

Literature on technocratic ideology and authority argues that technological domination incapacitates people by placing control of decisions about fundamental aspects of their lives in the hands of others. Knowledge and responsibility for action are taken out of laypersons' hands as they are rendered into passive objects of technocratic decision making. This critique of technocratic ideology, however, does not adequately incorporate gender as a category of inquiry. It does not fully portray how the logic of technology subordinates women in active social relations. In this study I have specified the social relations and technocratic ideology that characterize contemporary childbirth practices. In addition, I have assessed the consequences of efforts to establish childbirth practices which empower women.

The medical model of childbirth claims to be grounded in science and technology. It defines childbirth as a medical event requiring hospitalization, the attendance of a physician, and careful monitoring with high-technology devices and procedures. The body is equated with a machine, and the physician serves as its technician. Despite the fact that childbirth is an intimate event of great importance to the individuals involved, their experiences are sacrificed to "normalcy" and "risk" reduction. Each individual labor must conform to what is defined as normal by the profession of obstetrics. Deviations from the norm are defined as pathological and as requiring intervention with monitors, drugs, and, frequently, surgery. The medical model of childbirth is characterized by reliance on standard procedures, expert decision making, and technological apparatus, despite a lack of evidence that these lead to better birth outcomes.

Authority and expertise in childbirth and even the definition of the event are male dominated and embedded in gender issues. The authority of the physician over the patient has resulted in mistreatment of pregnant women by physicians and increasing subordination of women to fetuses. Interest in and attention toward the fetus often override that given to the mother, particularly as advanced technology has made it possible to gain more information about the health of the fetus *in utero*. Consequently, a major goal from a feminist perspective is the reappropriation of control over the birth process by women.

The midwifery approach is rooted in a different philosophy of birth and consequently leads to different practices. Birth is understood as something which women do, not something which is done to them. It is the birthing woman who gives birth while midwives offer support and assistance. This approach to birth reflects an understanding that birth is also an important event in families. Family members must be welcomed and included in the pregnancy and the birth. By giving credence to the experiential knowledge of women, the midwifery model offers a woman-centered approach to birth that affords birthing women much more autonomy and control over their birth experiences than the medical model does.

My analysis is rooted in ongoing participant observation of a free-standing birth center for more than ten years. I have worked as a volunteer at the center, have birthed two children as a client, and have served on the foundation board. I have been a supporter and a critical observer of the center, trying to secure its existence while at the same time maintaining enough critical distance to analyze its problems, its structural context, and its relationship to other birth options such as home birth.

When I began working on this project I did not intend to be involved with it for so long, nor could I foresee the many forms my involvement would take. Also, I imagined that I was researching and writing the beginning of a story that would continue for a long time. Now I fear I may actually be writing the end of the story as well. As the previous chapter indicates, the dwindling client base at the birth center raises questions about the center's ability to survive over the next several years. Anne Watson's deep commitment to the center will more than likely keep it going until her retirement, but there is no obvious person to take over for her. If the client base can be increased, it would probably be possible to find another nurse-midwife willing to take over the center. If the client base remains small and resources remain tight, there is little likelihood of a takeover, at least not by a nurse-midwife.

As mentioned earlier, a local hospital has been interested in taking over the birth center for years. Their intentions for the center are not clear. Mathews and Zadak (1991) report that some health industry consultants predict that more free-standing birth centers (FSBCs) will be owned and operated by physicians, although they will not necessarily provide the care in these centers. As such takeovers occur technologies now limited to hospitals are likely to find their way into FSBCs, rationalized through cost-effectiveness and safety concerns. Supporters of the birth center fear that if the local hospital did take over, everything would change. This small, personal facility run by nurse-midwives and supported by a community of women and families would become part of a much larger institution. Decision making would shift to physicians and to the hospital bureaucracy. The autonomy of birthing women would be severely compromised under such circumstances.

This case study began by analyzing two different attempts to establish a free-standing birth center. The effort on the part of Babyplace had little success in gaining support, while Anne Watson and her supporters were successful for several reasons. Because of Anne's previous employment at the medical center and her experience in operating a birth center in another state, she was able to provide the skillful leadership required to negotiate the complex process of establishing a birth center. The fact that she had medical credentials that were acceptable to at least some members of the medical establishment made it possible for her to get the backup support necessary for her to proceed with her plan.

The efforts of both Babyplace and Anne Watson can best be analyzed and understood in the context of the environment in which they were operating. The physician-dominated medical climate in the state is supported by the legal mechanisms which govern the practice of nurse-midwifery. The requirement that nurse-midwives practice in alliance with a physician gives physicians control over the types of childbirth alternatives which can be established and who can establish them. Anne Watson was able to acquire backup support because of her medical training and credentials and her previous experience as director of midwifery services at a birth center. Babyplace, however, was unable to acquire similar support. As consumers, they lacked the training and credentials necessary to be taken seriously by physicians. Their inability to enter into an alliance with a physician was the most serious obstacle to their success. The requirement of physician support demonstrates the power of the medical model and the need even for those who challenge this model to make connections with the medical establishment.

While the state health council stated its support for childbirth alternatives, it clearly favored those established and run by health professionals. The requirements established by the health council regarding property and financial resources made it impossible for Babyplace to even file a certificate of need, much less gain approval for their project. Anne Watson, on the other hand, received strong support from the health council. A birth center with a nurse-midwife as director fell directly in line with the health council's idea of what constituted a good childbirth alternative. The certificate of need filed by the nurse-midwife provided more than the information requested by the council and demonstrated the type of financial stability that the council required.

One of the important features of those active in support of the birth center has been their single-minded focus on establishing and maintaining the birth center. They have always defined their goal narrowly: to provide a safe, woman-centered alternative to the dominant form of obstetrics. Because they do not wish to link their goals to those of the larger women's health movement or to the women's movement generally, they have been careful to separate themselves from groups, such as feminist groups, which might be considered politically radical. Nor have the birth center supporters represented any clear-cut ideological position. Like birth center clients, they have spanned the political spectrum from left to right. This diversity makes it difficult to tie the birth center to a broader political agenda. There are supporters and clients who see the center as tied to a feminist agenda and those who see it as representing a rejection of just such an agenda. This reflects Rothman's (1982) observation about the home birth movement in the United States. Rothman argues that this movement represents an alliance between feminists and traditionalists. For feminists childbirth is one among many issues regarding the control which women have over their lives. For traditionalists the issue has to do with family involvement and control over birth.

Over the center's years of operation, the extent of its vulnerability to the medical model has become increasingly clear. Unexpected problems with third-party reimbursement and malpractice insurance have served to underline the need for the center to tailor its practices and its politics to be consistent with established medical standards. From the beginning, the nurse-midwives at the center have carefully screened out those patients defined by the medical model as high risk. Over the years, nurse-midwives have been forced to enact some slight changes in routine practice. For example, they are now required by law to use medication in the eyes of newborns to combat possible infection due to the presence of venereal disease in the vaginal tract. Prior to this legal requirement, the decision whether to use such medication was left to birthing women.

Establishment of the birth center has meant a significant change in childbirth options for women and families in the area. Women receive careful attention and are treated with respect. They are expected to take an active role in their own care during pregnancy and birth. Nurse-midwives serve as attendants at birth, intervening as little as possible during the birth process. Those who have received care and given birth at the birth center have expressed their overwhelming enthusiasm and support in response to their experience. At the same time, the clientele is a small percentage of the childbearing population in the area and represents no serious threat to the medical model. In fact, although the birth center provides an extremely important option for childbearing women, it serves as a safety valve which may actually protect the medical model.

When Anne Watson left the local medical center, a number of nurses who shared her commitment to patient advocacy and her ideas about birthing also left. This meant that a number of practitioners who might have challenged the ideas and practices of the medical model from inside the hospital were no longer part of the institution. Once the birth center was established, it provided a place for women dissatisfied with hospital birth to give birth elsewhere. Without the birth center, some of them would have given birth at home but most would have gone to the local medical center. It is possible that if the birth center did not provide an opportunity for out-of-hospital birthing, more pressure would have been brought to bear on the medical center to make more accommodations to the needs of birthing women.

Some accommodations have been made since the birth center's opening. The availability of a birthing room has been well received by consumers, and all women and families who go to the medical center have benefited from a more liberal policy that allows siblings to visit mothers and newborns shortly after birth. New labor-delivery-recovery rooms have recently opened, so that women no longer have to move from room to room while in active labor.

At the same time that these innovations continue to take place, birth at the medical center is not becoming any less technologically defined. The Cesarean section rate is 24 percent and the majority of women who give birth at the medical center receive epidural anesthesia. On a recent tour of the new maternity facilities, the nurse conducting the tour pointed out the wide, brightly lit hallways and expressed the hope that laboring women would walk them during labor. This would be possible, she said, because of the telemetric monitors, which can monitor women even as they are walking around the hospital. Anne Watson believes that it is not the concessions to woman-centered birthing which attract women to the medical center, but rather the dependence on technology and the availability of epidurals.

Anne's beliefs are consistent with Jordan's observations regarding the changes in birthing in the United States between the late 1970s and the early 1990s. Jordan expected that over time birth would become less technologized and more responsive to the needs of birthing women. What has happened instead is that births have become more medicalized and technologized and women have been socialized not only to accept but to expect the technocratic model of birth and the authority of the physician which this model implies (Jordan, 1993).

CONSTRAINED PROGRESS

As the preceding chapter demonstrates, the birth center exists within a structural context which supports the medical model. Free-standing birth centers and nurse-midwives who work in them struggle to carve out a niche in this context. On the one hand they challenge the assumptions and practices of the medical model. On the other hand they require the recognition and support of the legal and financial institutions which support the medical model.

The case study presented here demonstrates a pattern of relations between the birth center and the medical model. Certain features of the medical model are also characteristic of the birth center, including affirmations of the legal control of birth practices and beliefs in expertise as demonstrated by licensure and certification. Beyond this, the birth center accommodates its practices to the demands of the medical model as required by law and by professional hierarchies. Nurse-midwives practicing at the center carefully screen clients as to their eligibility for birth center care, using criteria developed by the profession of obstetrics for categorizing high-risk pregnancies. On the other hand, the birth center affirms core beliefs that are in opposition to those which underlie the medical model. The philosophy upon which the center is based sees pregnancy and birth as healthy processes that do not routinely require medical or technological intervention. Pregnancy and birth are woman-centered events during which women are expected to act as responsible and knowledgeable participants in their own care.

The beliefs around which the dominant model and the birth center converge, as well as the demands of the dominant model to which the birth center alternative accommodates, can be viewed as expressions of patriarchal discourse and power. Legal rationality, professional hierarchy, and economic rationality give primacy to objectivism, emotional detachment, and technical calculation (Fee, 1983; Harding, 1986; Rothman, 1989). These orientations facilitate administrative power and the interests of the medical establishment through technical and rule-ordered discourse. The beliefs that the birth center holds in opposition to the dominant model can be viewed as central to feminism. Intimacy, emotional involvement, responsible participation, and a sharing of practical and technical knowledge are core features of the woman-centered philosophy which guides the center.

In the everyday practice of the birth center, these patriarchal and feminist beliefs are generally isolated from one another. This is bolstered by the fact that birth center supporters do not try to establish a shared political vision or a broader philosophical purpose. The nature of care at the center and the interactions between practitioners and clients are guided by woman-centered values. People engaged in both receiving and giving care are focused on their immediate interactions and not on the ideological and political context in which they are operating. Indeed, although birth center participants may disagree deeply about the location and meaning of birth in a larger political agenda, they share a belief about the importance of the experience of birth for women and families.

At the same time, these patriarchal and feminist beliefs are contradictory at the level of forming a politics around birth alternatives. The contradictions between these beliefs are manifested in the public discourse and public presentation of the birth center. Arguments by spokespersons for the center concerning the need for this alternative typically focus on consumer demand, choice maximization, and cost-effectiveness. Instead of expressing the woman-centered values that guide practice, public discourse has been rooted largely in the rationality of the dominant model.

As the previous chapter pointed out, the foundation board intends to take a somewhat broader approach than they have in the past to generate support for, and to increase the client base of, the birth center. The board has indicated its desire to seek ties to other health-oriented groups in the area and possibly to network with those involved with home birth.

REAPPROPRIATING BIRTH: SHORT-TERM AND LONG-TERM GOALS

The power of established medical interests and of the institutional context which supports them creates a difficult terrain for woman-centered birthing. Dominant medical practices and patriarchal thinking dominate the public discourse over birth. Even the public discourse over the birth center, which in many ways challenges the medical model, is centered around questions of safety, cost, and family interests. If the goal is to reappropriate control of birthing by women, the constraints imposed by the medical model on birth centers and even on home birth create strategic dilemmas. One way to get beyond these is to distinguish between short-term and long-term outcomes and try to pursue both strategies simultaneously.

In the short term it is important to support and expand out-of-hospital birthing options such as free-standing birth centers, even though the medical model continues to dominate. The establishment and operation of the birth center demonstrate that some latitude exists within the structural context which supports the medical model. On the other hand, the problems which the birth center has experienced demonstrate the power of established medical interests and the vulnerability of the birth center within that context. At the same time that the birth center has encountered problems, other birth centers around the country have closed their doors. Currently only about 130 centers exist nationwide, down from more than 200 in the late 1980s. There are, however, about 90 centers in the process of opening.

Although the birth center is vulnerable in a number of ways, some positive changes which have occurred over its years of operation have helped the center to remain viable. The passage of state legislation mandating third-party reimbursement was important for nurse-midwives as well as for birth center clients. It insures that neither insurance companies nor employers can discriminate against nurse-midwives.

A second policy change was the recent approval of the birth center for Medicaid reimbursement. During the center's first few years of operation, it was Medicaid policy in the state to reimburse nurse-midwives but not birth center facilities. Now that the birth center itself has been approved for reimbursement, it can accept Medicaid clients. At the present time, however, not many Medicaid recipients find their way to the birth center. Some type of outreach program is necessary to inform these potential clients of the center's existence and the prenatal and birthing services it provides. Anne Watson, however, faces a dilemma regarding Medicaid clients, given the present size of the birth center clientele. It is important to increase the size of that clientele, but the amount of the Medicaid reimbursement does not cover the cost of the services provided. Before any concentrated effort can be made to bring more Medicaid clients to the center, the overall size of the general clientele needs to increase.

A third change of importance to nurse-midwives came when advanced practice nursing legislation was signed into law in the summer of 1994. Although not specific to nurse-midwives, this legislation is relevant to their practice. Most notably, it gives them the authority to prescribe medication. These policy changes have improved conditions for nurse-midwives in the state by making it somewhat easier for them to establish practices and by making their employment more secure.

Another change which would improve the situation still more would be the repeal of the law requiring nurse-midwives to establish an alliance with a physician in order to practice. If the legal requirement is to stand, the state should have the burden of locating physicians to work in alliance with nurse-midwives. At present, written evidence of collaboration is required in about half of the states, and in the others it is expected that midwives will practice in collaboration with a physician who can be called in if physician backup is required. Such arrangements often work well and can help to make the care of pregnant and birthing women go smoothly no matter what contingencies develop. A well-established alliance can assure a smooth transition from birth center to hospital if an emergency should arise. The current law, however, gives physicians the power to determine whether or not nurse-midwives can practice in the state and makes nurse-midwives completely vulnerable to the authority of the medical establishment.

While short-term policy changes are important, there are also broader political and ideological issues that need to be considered. As has been pointed out, there is an absence of political consensus among birth center activists and clients, as well as a conflict between the values which shape birth practices at the center and the public presentation of the center. The resulting absence of a coherent political viewpoint becomes more significant as constraints imposed by the medical model become more severe and a qualitative change in the degree of subordination of women to the welfare of fetuses takes place.

Despite the availability of midwives, birth centers, and home birth, research indicates that dominant ideology and practice surrounding childbirth (and reproduction generally) are becoming more authoritarian, male centered, and technological. While a minority of women and families reject the medical model in favor of woman-centered birthing, the majority of women continue to give birth in accordance with that model. which is becoming more, not less, technological (Jordan, 1993; Davis-Floyd, 1992; Rothman, 1989).

Currently, nearly one out of every four births is a Cesarean section despite a consensus between physicians and critics that this figure is too high and represents a great many unnecessary surgeries. In fact, the number of court-ordered Cesarean sections is likely to increase. The use of ultrasound to monitor the growth and condition of the fetus *in utero* is becoming a standard part of treatment during pregnancy. The development of reproductive technologies such as embryo transfer and *in vitro* fertilization is changing the way that reproduction takes place and redefining the role of women in reproduction (Stanworth, 1988; Spallone and Steinberg, 1987). Increasing attention is being paid to the fetus as more information can be gathered through diagnostic procedures such as amniocentesis and chorionic villus sampling. In recent years there have been several cases of brain-dead pregnant women being artificially kept alive long enough to be delivered (Corea, 1985b). The popular image of reproduction is of something which requires technology to be accomplished and in which the role of women is secondary, at best, to that of machinery and medical experts. In Davis-Floyd's words, birth becomes a "technocratic service that obstetrics supplies to society" (1992, p. 57). Giving birth is not merely a biological function. Rather, it is an experience which is culturally shaped and determined. The more reproduction is subject to technological definitions and procedures, the more difficult it will be for women to reject the dominant model in favor of more empowering alternatives.

The emergence of birth centers is an extremely promising development, and the types of policy changes discussed above would facilitate the practice of nurse-midwifery in the birth center setting. It is important, however, not to lose sight of the larger context within which birth centers are located. Currently, every aspect of reproduction from conception through birth is being redefined in response to reproductive technologies which not only objectify women but which also seriously call into question the whole nature of biological motherhood (Corea, 1985b; Rothman, 1989; Spallone and Steinberg, 1987; Stanworth, 1988). Increasingly, for example, women are being referred to as one possible "maternal environment."

Technologies reflect and reinforce the social relations and knowledge that give rise to them. Race, class, and gender inequalities are therefore enhanced by current developments in reproductive technologies. It is clear that the birth center movement must become part of larger feminist efforts to insure women's reproductive rights and women's rights more generally. These efforts have the potential to provide the basis for the public articulation of the values which underlie the everyday practice of nurse-midwifery, such as those found in the birth center analyzed in this study. At this point in history, the growth of birth practices which are empowering for women can best be accomplished through political and social movements with a fuller feminist agenda. Otherwise, such options will remain tiny enclaves within a medical model which moves toward a greater and greater subordination of women and which continually becomes more invasive.

In the discussion of the midwifery model in Chapter 4 I talk about Rothman's (1989) argument that a feminist agenda for birthing must focus on empowering midwives so that they can be fully autonomous professionals not controlled by physicians. Doing so requires challenging the definition of childbirth as a medical event. If childbirth were seen as more than a medical event, the medical profession could no longer exercise a near monopoly over birth. As fully autonomous professionals, midwives would set the standards for the practice of midwifery and could advise the state on the licensing of midwives.

Certainly these changes would significantly alter conditions for all midwives, regardless of the settings in which they practice. They would definitely be important for the birth center with which this study is concerned.

THE IMPORTANCE OF THE BIRTH CENTER FOR WOMEN AND FAMILIES

Rothman (1989) argues that woman-taught, woman-controlled midwifery is feminist praxis, meaning that midwives work with the labor of women to shape the birth experience to meet the needs of women. She is quick to distinguish between such midwives and the medically trained nurse-specialists who call themselves nurse-midwives. Rothman argues that some nurse-midwives are part of the midwifery tradition while others are not.

I believe that Anne Watson and most of the other nurse-midwives who have worked at the birth center over the years of its operation are very much a part of the midwifery tradition. They publicly self-identify with it and with its rich history.

At a public lecture given at a local university, Anne once described an experience that she had shortly after becoming a nurse-midwife. She was being considered for a position at a major hospital in a large urban center and was invited to tour their obstetrical facilities. At one point she was taken into a large room where several laboring women were lying in troughlike beds with football helmets on their heads. The beds and helmets were to protect the women from injury which might result from any flailing brought on by drugs given during labor. Anne's reaction was that she would never be a part of such treatment of women. She left the hospital and went to work for a home birth service primarily for low-income women.

During Anne's career she has practiced nurse-midwifery in a variety of settings, at home, in a hospital, and in free-standing birth centers. In every setting she has acted as an advocate for women, frequently at great personal cost. In public lectures she describes the philosophy which shapes her relationship with the women she assists as one of mutual respect. She always urges women to empower themselves with regard to their own health care and consistently speaks of the need for birth settings and practices which empower women.

In addition to hearing her words, I have had the privilege of observing her activities over the past twelve years. I have seen her with pregnant women, with new families, with past clients who come back to renew the important bond that they formed with her when she assisted them through pregnancies and births. I have experienced her care and compassion directly. She has been with me through one of the most difficult and two of the happiest times of my life. She has provided care, nurturance, respect, and support to all of the women and families who have come to the birth center over its years of operation. One of Anne's backup physicians has said that Anne has made more of an impact on obstetrical care in the state in which she practices than anyone else. There is no doubt that the work that Anne has done through her advocacy for women birthing in the hospital and through establishing the birth center has had a lasting impact on the experiences of birthing women and their families.

Nurse-midwifery care at the birth center is woman-centered, and great importance is given to the experiential knowledge of birthing women. The nurse-midwives demonstrate a respect for and a confidence in the ability of women to birth without interference. They see birth as an important event in the lives of women and families, and they welcome families to be part of pregnancy and birth. They invite women to shape their pregnancy and birth experiences to meet their own needs and desires.

Rothman (1983) argues that free-standing birth centers represent a compromise between client and practitioner needs. Birth centers meet the needs of nurse-midwifery as a profession, offering more autonomy for nurse-midwives than the hospital setting. They also meet the needs of individual nurse-midwives, overcoming the problems of a home birth practice where one might be constantly on call and sometimes have two clients in labor at the same time. However, the autonomy which free-standing birth centers offer is limited by the features of the structural context which have been discussed. Also, FSBCs may not overcome all the potential problems of a home birth practice. The fact that clients come to the center means the individual nurse-midwives do not face the problem of having to be in two places at once if two clients go into labor at the same time. But nurse-midwives working in birth centers may, like home birth practitioners, find themselves on call most of the time. This has been true for Anne as the number of birth center clients has dropped to a level which can no longer support two or more full-time nurse-midwives.

Rothman (1983) argues that birth centers reinforce the belief that birth needs to occur in some "special place" removed from the "mainstream of life." For people who view birth in this way birth centers are acceptable. They do not, however, meet the needs of those who see birth as a healthy process and who want to integrate it into family life.

It is certainly true that not all women who reject the medical model of birth find birth centers acceptable. Some women want to give birth at home and see no reason to do otherwise. In interviews that I have done with women who have given birth at home, there were some who wanted to do so and who sought out a midwife who would assist them. They never considered a birth center birth. Other women did not want a hospital birth and looked into the possibility of birthing at the birth center, but did not meet the low-risk criteria. In two of these cases, the women were pregnant with twins. One of these women had had a previous Cesarean section. The birth center refers twin pregnancies to the care of the backup physicians and transfers women having vaginal births after a Cesarean to the hospital. Neither of these women would agree to birth in the hospital. Both gave birth to healthy twins at home.

Yet there are women, myself included, who do not believe that birth requires a special place but who choose the birth center for other reasons. Many women who know Anne want her to care for them through their pregnancies. Women and families become attached not only to Anne and to the other nurse-midwives and nurses at the center, but also to the center itself. Women come there for all their prenatal care. By the time they are ready to give birth they feel comfortable at the birth center. They are familiar with the feel of the place, its sounds, and its smells. Many women remark about the wonderful smell of the birth center and how the memory of it stays with them long after their births.

The birth center is not an institutional setting like a clinic or a hospital. It is a place that is in large part shaped by the people who use it. Anne often reminds clients, "It is your birth center." Indeed, the center bears the marks of many women who have labored and birthed their children there. As mentioned in an earlier chapter, many clients donate artwork, furniture, supplies, or books. Many others become active around the politics of the birth center and donate time and effort toward maintaining the center.

It is not only birthing women who are touched by the birth center's existence. It is also important in the lives of their families and friends. I go to the birth center often for meetings and gatherings. Frequently my four-year-old daughter goes with me. Before we leave the center, we always have to make a stop at the room where she was born. If others are around, she asks them to come see her special room. It is always a lovely moment because it leads to a sharing of the special memories of other babies born in the room and in the other rooms that make up this wonderful place. The birth center is not home but it is much more than a building where women and families come to have babies. It is the center of a community of women and families who, despite major political differences, share a commitment to this way of birth and to challenging the medical model.

There are certainly women who come to the birth center who would not consider home birth. Indeed, this is true of the majority of birth center clients. One reason birth centers are so important is that they offer an out-of-hospital birth experience, relatively free from intervention, to a population of women and families who would otherwise, for the most part, birth in the hospital. Through their birth center experience they come to see birth in a different way. Very few women who give birth at the birth center go to the hospital for subsequent births. Most return to the center, and a few have home births.

The philosophy and practice at the birth center pose a significant challenge to the technocratic practices of the medical model. The problem faced by this birth center and others is that they are embedded within the very model they challenge and therefore remain constrained by it and vulnerable to it. The context is complex and contradictory. At the same time that there are factors which threaten the birth center, there are others which actually facilitate its existence. There is no question that strengthening the autonomy of nurse-midwives, and midwives generally, would lessen the vulnerability of birth centers and would help insure that the birthing experiences they offer remain available for women and families.

Bibliography

Alchon, Guy. 1985. *The Invisible Hand of Planning*. Princeton, N.J.: Princeton University Press.

Annandale, Ellen C. 1988. "How Midwives Accomplish Natural Birth: Managing Risk and Balancing Expectations." *Social Problems* 35, no. 2 (April): 95–109.

Arditti, Rita, Renate Duelli Klein, and Shelley Minden. 1984. *Test-Tube Women: What Future for Motherhood?* London: Pandora Press.

Arms, Suzanne. 1975. *Immaculate Deception*. New York: Bantam Books.

Arney, William Ray. 1982. *Power and the Profession of Obstetrics*. Chicago: University of Chicago Press.

Ashford, Janet Isaacs. 1983. *The Wholebirth Catalog*. Trumansburg, N.Y.: Crossing Press.

———.1985. "Risks of Epidural Anesthesia." *Childbirth Alternatives Quarterly* 6, no. 3 (spring).

———.1986. "Midwifery on Trial Again." *Childbirth Alternatives Quarterly* 8, no.2 (winter).

———.1986–87. "The Pamela Stewart Case." *Childbirth Alternatives Quarterly* (winter).

Banta, H. David, and Stephen B. Thacker. 1979. *Costs and Benefits of Electronic Fetal Monitoring: A Review of the Literature*. National Center for Health Services Research (NCHSR), Research Report Series, U.S. Department of Health, Education, and Welfare, April 1979.

Barker-Benfield, G. J. 1976. *Horrors of the Half-Known Life*. New York: Harper Colophon Books.

Bell, Daniel. 1967. "The Year 2000: The Trajectory of an Idea." *Daedalus* 96, no. 3 (summer).

Berman, Daniel M. 1978. *Death on the Job: Occupational Health and Safety Struggles in the United States*. New York: Monthly Review Press.

Bernstein, Patricia. 1993. *Having a Baby: Mothers Tell Their Stories*. New York: Pocket Books.

Bidgood-Wilson, Mary, Carol Barickman, and Susan Ackley. 1992. "Nurse-Midwifery Today: A Legislative Update." Parts 1 and 2. *Journal of Nurse-Midwifery* 37, no. 2 (March/April); no. 3 (May/June).

Bleier, Ruth. 1984. *Science and Gender: A Critique of Biology and Its Theories on Women*. New York: Pergamon Press.

Braverman, Harry. 1974. *Labor and Monopoly Capital: The Degradation of Work in the Twentieth Century.* New York: Monthly Review Press.

Broomfield, John H. 1980. "High Technology: The Construction of Disaster." *Alternative Futures* 3, no. 2.

Cockburn, Cynthia. 1992. "The Circuit of Technology: Gender, Identity, and Power." In *Consuming Technologies: Media and Information in Domestic Spaces,* edited by Roger Silverstone and Eric Hirsch. London: Routledge.

Collins, Patricia Hill. 1986. "Learning from the Outsider Within: The Sociological Significance of Black Feminist Thought." *Social Problems* 33, no. 6 (December).

Corea, Gena. 1985a. *The Hidden Malpractice.* Rev. ed. New York: Harper and Row.

——— .1985b. *The Mother Machine: Reproductive Technologies from Artificial Insemination to Artificial Wombs.* New York: Harper and Row.

Cosminsky, Sheila. 1982. "Childbirth and Change: A Guatemalan Study." In *Ethnography of Fertility and Birth,* edited by Carol R. MacCormack. London: Academic Press.

Davis-Floyd, Robbie. 1987. "Obstetric Training as a Rite of Passage." *Medical Anthropology Quarterly* 1, no. 3 (September).

——— .1992. *Birth as an American Rite of Passage.* Berkeley: University of California Press.

DeVries, Raymond G. 1985. *Regulating Birth: Midwives, Medicine and the Law.* Philadelphia: Temple University Press.

Dickson, David. 1981. "Limiting Democracy: Technocrats and the Liberal State." *Democracy* (January).

——— .1984. *The New Politics of Science.* New York: Pantheon Books.

Duden, Barbara. 1993. *Disembodying Women: Perspectives on Pregnancy and the Unborn.* Translated by Lee Hornacki. Cambridge: Harvard University Press.

Dwinnell, Jane. 1992. *Birth Stories: Mystery, Power, and Creation.* Westport, Conn.: Bergin and Garvey.

Eakins, Pamela S. 1986a. "The American Way of Birth." in *The American Way of Birth,* edited by Pamela S. Eakins. Philadelphia: Temple University Press.

——— .1986b. "Out-of-Hospital Birth." In *The American Way of Birth,* edited by Pamela S. Eakins. Philadelphia: Temple University Press.

Edwards, Margot, and Mary Waldorf. 1984. *Reclaiming Birth: History and Heroines of American Childbirth Reform.* Trumansburg, N.Y.: Crossing Press.

Ehrenreich, Barbara, and Deirdre English. 1979. *For Her Own Good: 150 Years of the Experts' Advice to Women.* Garden City, N.Y.: Anchor Books.

Ellul, Jacques. 1964. *Technological Society.* New York: Alfred A. Knopf.

Ernst, Eunice K. M. 1985. "NACC Presentation at ICEA/NIH [International Childbirth Education Association/National Institutes of Health] Forum" *NACC News* (National Association of Childbearing Centers, Perkiomenville, Penn.) fall.

Ettner, Frederick. 1977. "Hospital Technology Breeds Pathology." *Women and Health* (September/October).

Fee, Elizabeth. 1983. "Women's Nature and Scientific Expertise." In *Women's Nature: Rationalizations of Inequality,* edited by Ruth Hubbard and Marion Lowe. New York: Pergamon Press.

Firestone, Shulamith. 1971. *The Dialectic of Sex.* London: Paladin.

Fishel, Leslie H., Jr. 1967. "The Problem of Social Control." In *Technology in Western Civilization,* edited by Melvin Kranzberg and Caroll W. Pursell, Jr. New York: Oxford University Press.

Florman, Samuel C. 1980. "Technology and the Tragic View." *Alternative Futures* 3, no. 2.

————. 1981. *Blaming Technology: The Irrational Search for Scapegoats.* New York: St. Martin's Press.

Foucault, Michel. 1973. *Birth of the Clinic.* New York: Pantheon Books.

————.1977. *Power/Knowledge: Selected Interviews and Other Writings.* Edited by Colin Gordon. New York: Pantheon Books.

Friedman, John. 1973. *Retracking America.* New York: Doubleday.

Fuller, R. Buckminster. 1969. *Utopia or Oblivion: The Prospects for Humanity.* New York: Overlook Press.

Gallagher, Janet. 1984. "The Fetus and the Law—Whose Life Is It Anyway?" *Ms.,* September.

Gaskin, Ina May. 1978. *Spiritual Midwifery.* Summertown, Tenn.: The Book Publishing Company.

Gilgoff, Anne. 1978. *Home Birth.* New York: Coward, McCann, and Geoghegan.

Guthman, Edwin. 1981. "Charlotte Observer Hunted a Killer in the Carolinas." *Philadelphia Inquirer,* April 19, 7–G.

Habermas, Jurgen,1971. *Knowledge and Human Interests.* Boston: Beacon Press.

————.1973. *Legitimation Crisis.* Boston: Beacon Press.

Harding, Sandra. 1986. *The Science Question in Feminism.* Ithaca, N.Y.: Cornell University Press.

Harrington, Michael. 1984. *The New American Poverty.* New York: Penguin Books.

Harrison, Michelle. 1982. *A Woman in Residence.* New York: Random House.

Hartouni, Valerie. 1991. "Containing Women: Reproductive Discourse in the 1980s." In *Technoculture,* edited by Constance Penley and Andres Ross. Minneapolis: University of Minnesota Press.

Haverkamp, Albert D., Miriam Orlean, Sharon Langendoerfer, John McFee, James Murphy, and Horace E. Thompson. 1979. "A Controlled Trial of Differential Effects of Intrapartum Monitoring." *American Journal of Obstetrics and Gynecology* 134, no. 4 (June 15).

Haverkamp, Albert D., Horace E. Thompson, John G. McFee, and Curtis Cetrulo. 1976. "The Evaluation of Continuous Heart Rate Monitoring in High-Risk Pregnancy." *American Journal of Obstetrics and Gynecology* 125, no. 3 (June 1).

Hubbard, Ruth. 1984. "Personal Courage Is Not Enough." In *Test-Tube Women: What Future for Motherhood?* edited by Rita Arditti, Renate Duelli-Klein, and Shelley Minden. London: Pandora Press.

Illich, Ivan. 1976. *Medical Nemesis: The Expropriation of Health.* New York: Pantheon Books.

Ingersoll, David, and Daniel Rich. 1978. "The One Dimensional Future." *Alternative Futures* 1, no. 1.

Jordan, Brigitte. 1980. *Birth in Four Cultures.* Montreal: Eden Press Women's Publications.

————. 1984. "External Cephalic Version as an Alternative to Breech Delivery and Cesarean Section." *Social Science and Medicine* 18, no. 8.

————. 1993. *Birth in Four Cultures.* 4th ed., revised and expanded by Robbie Davis-Floyd. Prospect Heights, Ill.: Waveland Press.

Kahn, Herman, and Anthony J. Weiner. 1967. "The Next Thirty Years: A Framework for Speculation." *Daedalus* (summer).

Kazis, Richard, and Richard L. Grossman. 1982. *Fear at Work: Job Blackmail, Labor, and the Environment.* New York: Pilgrim Press.

Keller, Evelyn Fox. 1985. *Reflections on Gender and Science*. New Haven, Conn.: Yale University Press.

Kelly, John. 1979. "Baby '79: Childbirth Today." *Ladies Home Journal*, January.

Kitzinger, Sheila, ed., 1988. *The Midwife Challenge*. London: Pandora Press.

Klee, Linea. 1986. "Home Away from Home: The Alternative Birth Center." *Social Science and Medicine* 23, no. 1: 9–16.

Kranzberg, Melvin. 1980. "Technology: The Half-Full Cup." *Alternative Futures*, special issue on Technology and Pessimism (spring).

Laderman, Carol. 1983. *Wives and Midwives: Childbirth and Nutrition in Rural Malaysia*. Berkeley: University of California Press.

Lagercrantz, Hugo, and Theodore A. Slotkin. 1986. "The Stress of Being Born." *Scientific American* (April).

Leavitt, Judith Walzer. 1986. *Brought to Bed: Childbearing in America, 1750–1950*. New York: Oxford University Press.

Lubic, Ruth Watson. 1981. "Alternative Maternity Care: Resistance and Change." In *Childbirth: Alternatives to Medical Control*, edited by Shelly Romalis. Austin: University of Texas Press.

Marcuse, Herbert. 1964. *One-Dimensional Man: Studies in the Ideology of Advanced Industrial Society*. Boston: Beacon Press.

Margolin, Steven. 1974. "What Do Bosses Do?: The Origins and Functions of Hierarchy in Capitalist Production." *Review of Radical Political Economics* (summer).

Martin, Emily. 1984. "Pregnancy, Labor, and Body Image in the United States." *Social Science and Medicine* 19, no. 11.

——— . 1987. *The Woman in the Body*. Boston: Beacon Press.

Martin, Gwen. 1994. "Selling My Eggs." *Glamour*, May, 168.

Mathews, Joan J., and Kathleen Zadak. 1991. "The Alternative Birth Movement in the United States: History and Current Status." *Women and Health* 17, no. 1.

Maurin, Judith. 1980. "Negotiating an Innovative Health Care Service." *Research in the Sociology of Health Care* 1.

Mehl, Lewis. 1978. "The Outcome of Home Delivery in the United States." In *The Place of Birth*, edited by Sheila Kitzinger and John A. Davis. Oxford: Oxford University Press.

Mendolsohn, Robert S. 1976. "Childbirth Alternatives and Infant Outcome: A Pediatric View." In *Safe Alternatives in Childbirth*, edited by David Stewart and Lee Stewart. Chapel Hill, N.C.: National Association of Parents and Professionals for Safe Alternatives in Childbirth.

Morgall, Janine. 1993. *Technology Assessment: A Feminist Perspective*. Philadelphia: Temple University Press.

Mumford, Lewis. 1972. "Authoritarian and Democratic Technics." In *Technology and Culture*, edited by Melvin Kranzberg and William H. Davenport. New York: Schocken Books.

Myers-Ciecko, Joanne. 1988. "Direct-Entry Midwifery in the USA." In *The Midwife Challenge*, edited by Sheila Kitzinger. London: Pandora Press.

NACC News (National Association of Childbearing Centers, Perkiomenville, Penn.). 1984–85. Vol. 2, nos. 3 and 4 (fall/winter).

Nelson, Margaret K. 1986. "Birth and Social Class." In *The American Way of Birth*, edited by Pamela S. Eakins. Philadelphia: Temple University Press.

Noble, David. 1977. *American by Design*. Oxford: Oxford University Press.

Oakley, Ann. 1984. *The Captured Womb: A History of the Medical Care of Pregnant Women*. Oxford: Basil Blackwell.

———. 1986. "Feminism, Motherhood, and Medicine—Who Cares?" In *What Is Feminism?* edited by Juliet Mitchell and Ann Oakley. New York: Pantheon Books.

Oakley, Ann, and Susanne Houd. 1990. *Helpers in Childbirth: Midwifery Today*. New York: Hemisphere Publishing.

Page, Joseph, and Mary-Win O'Brien. 1973. *Bitter Wages*. New York: Grossman Publishers.

Page, Lesley. 1988. "The Midwife's Role in Modern Health Care." In *The Midwife Challenge*, edited by Sheila Kitzinger. London: Pandora Press.

Palmer, Gabrielle. 1988. *The Politics of Breastfeeding*. London: Pandora Press.

Pascarella, Perry. 1979. *Technology: Fire in a Dark World*. New York: Van Nostrand Reinhold.

Price, Don K. 1965. *The Scientific Estate*. Cambridge: Harvard University Press.

Public Citizen Health Research Group. 1994. "Unnecessary Cesarean Sections: Curing a National Epidemic." *Health Letter* 10, no. 6 (June).

Rich, Adrienne. 1986. *Of Woman Born: Motherhood as Experience and Institution*. New York: W. W. Norton.

Rooks, Judith P., Norman L. Weatherby, Eunice K. M. Ernst, Susan Stapleton, David Rosen, and Allan Rosenfield. 1989. "Outcomes of Care in Birth Centers: The National Birth Center Study." *New England Journal of Medicine* 321 (December 28): 1804–1811.

Rothman, Barbara Katz. 1982. *In Labor: Women and Power in the Birthplace*. New York: W. W. Norton.

———. 1983. "Anatomy of a Compromise: Nurse-Midwifery and the Rise of the Birth Center." *Journal of Nurse-Midwifery* 28, no. 4 (July/August): 3–7.

———. 1989. *Recreating Motherhood: Ideology and Technology in Patriarchal Society*. New York: W. W. Norton.

Rowland, Robin. 1987. "Technology and Motherhood: Reproduction Choice Reconsidered." *Signs: Journal of Women in Culture and Society* 12, no. 3.

Ruddick, Sara. 1989. *Maternal Thinking: Toward a Politics of Peace*. Boston: Beacon Press.

Ruzek, Sheryl Burt. 1980. "Medical Response to Women's Health Activities: Conflict, Accommodation and Cooptation." *Research in the Sociology of Health Care* 1: 335–354.

———. 1993. "Defining Reducible Risk: Social Dimensions of Assessing Birth Technologies." *Human Nature* 4, no. 4 (May): 383–408.

Sallomi, Pacia, Angie Pallow-Fleury, and Peggy McMahon. 1982. *Midwifery and the Law*. Albuquerque, N.M.: Mothering Publications.

Sargent, Carolyn Fishel. 1982. *The Cultural Context of Therapeutic Choice*. Boston: D. Reidel Publishing.

Schon, Donald A. 1971. *Beyond the Stable State*. New York: W. W. Norton.

Shaw, Nancy Stoller. 1974. *Forced Labor: Maternity Care in the United States*. New York: Pergamon Press.

Shy, Kirkwood K., David Luthy, Forrest Bennett, Michael Whitfield, Eric Larson, Gerald van Belle, James P. Hughes, Judith A. Wilson, Morton A. Stenchever. 1990. "Effects of Electronic Fetal-Heart-Rate Monitoring, as Compared with Periodic Auscultation, on the Neurologic Development of Premature Infants." *New England Journal of Medicine* 322, no. 9 (March 1): 588–593.

Skinner, B. F. 1971. *Beyond Freedom and Dignity*. New York: Knopf.

Spallone, Patricia, and Deborah Lynn Steinberg. 1987. *Made to Order: The Myth of Reproductive and Genetic Progress*. New York: Pergamon Press.

Speert, Harold. 1979. *Obstetrics and Gynecology in America: A History*. Chicago: American College of Obstetricians and Gynecologists.

Stanworth, Michelle. 1988. *Reproductive Technologies: Gender, Motherhood and Medicine*. Minneapolis: University of Minnesota Press.

Starr, Paul. 1982. *The Social Transformation of American Medicine*. New York: Basic Books.

Sterling, Theodore. 1978. "Does Smoking Kill Workers or Working Kill Smokers? The Mutual Relationship Between Smoking, Occupation, and Respiratory Disease." *International Journal of Health Services* 8, no. 3.

Stewart, David, and Lee Stewart. 1976. *Safe Alternatives in Childbirth*. Chapel Hill, N.C.: National Association of Parents and Professionals for Safe Alternatives in Childbirth.

Stromberg, Ann Helton. 1988. "Women in Female-Dominated Professions." In *Women Working: Theories and Facts in Perspective*, edited by Ann Helton Stromberg and Shirley Harkess. Mountain View, Calif.: Mayfield Publishing.

Sullivan, Deborah, and Rose Weitz. 1988. *Labor Pains: Modern Midwives and Home Birth*. New Haven, Conn.: Yale University Press.

Teasley, Regi L. 1986. "Nurse and Lay Midwifery in Vermont." In *The American Way of Birth*, edited by Pamela S. Eakins. Philadelphia: Temple University Press.

Tew, Marjorie. 1990. *Safer Childbirth? A Critical History of Maternity Care*. London: Chapman and Hall.

Thompson, William Irwin. 1971. *At the Edge of History*. New York: Harper and Row.

Weitz, Rose, and Deborah A. Sullivan. 1986. "The Politics of Childbirth: The Re-emergence of Midwifery in Arizona." *Social Problems* 33, no. 3 (February).

Wertz, Richard W., and Dorothy C. Wertz. 1977. *Lying-In: A History of Childbirth in America*. New York: Free Press.

Whitehouse, Franklin. 1981. "Battle Is Joined Over 'Home Birthing.'" *New York Times*, December 2, A1.

Winner, Langdon. 1977. *Autonomous Technology: Technics Out-of-Control*. Cambridge: MIT Press.

——. 1986. *The Whale and the Reactor*. Chicago: University of Chicago Press.

Wolin, Sheldon S. 1981. "The New Public Philosophy." *Democracy* 1, no. 4 (October).

Women's Rights Law Reporter. 1982. "Reproductive Rights" (Symposium issue). Vol. 7, no. 3 (spring).

Index

ABOUT THE AUTHOR

KATHLEEN DOHERTY TURKEL is Assistant Professor in the Women's Studies Program at the University of Delaware. She teaches courses on motherhood in culture and politics and is a community activist supporting birth centers and creating favorable conditions for midwives.

ISBN 0-89789-317-4

EAN

HARDCOVER BAR CODE